KATHY SMITH'S
WINNING WORKOUT

12 WEEKS TO A BETTER BODY USING FREE WEIGHTS

BY KATHY SMITH with JUDY JONES

Running Press
Philadelphia, Pennsylvania

Canadian representatives: General Publishing Co., Ltd., 30 Lesmill Road, Don Mills, Ontario M3B 2T6.

International representatives: Worldwide Media Services, Inc., 115 East 23rd Street, New York, NY 10010.

9   8   7   6   5   4   3   2   1
Digit on the right indicates the number of this printing.

Library of Congress Cataloging-in-Publication Data
Smith, Kathy.
   Kathy Smith's winning workout.

   1. Physical fitness for women. 2. Exercise
for women. I. Jones, Judy. II. Title.
GV482.S64   1987   613.7'045   87-4554

ISBN 0-89471-529-1 cloth

Front jacket photograph by Dick Zimmerman
Back jacket photograph by Phillip Vullo
Cover design by Toby Schmidt
Interior photographs by Phillip Vullo
Typography: Goudy Oldstyle by Deputy Crown and Dynamo by Letraset
*Printed by Port City Press, Baltimore, MD. Bound by Short Run Bindery, Medford, NJ. Dust jacket printed by
Spectracolor-Reynolds, Cherry Hill, NJ.*

This book may be ordered by mail from the publisher.
Please include $1.50 for postage.
But try your bookstore first!
Running Press Book Publishers, 125 South 22nd Street, Philadelphia, Pennsylvania 19103

Contents

To Mom
For all her T.L.C.

My special thanks to Johnnie Ward, who has
been instrumental in the continued success of
the IN'TONE line, and to Mr. Curry, whom I
admire not only for his love of the industry,
but also for his scrupulous eye.

Introduction

There's been a virtual revolution in the exercise field over the last few years. Instead of the scattershot, any-exercise-is-better-than-no-exercise-at-all mentality that prevailed at the start of the fitness boom, we now take a more scientific approach to the business of getting and staying fit.

New technology and more sophisticated research, especially research in the training of top athletes, has enabled experts to distinguish the exercises that really work from those that just waste time, the safe activities from those that put too much strain on the body, and the factors that make it fun to stick to a fitness program from those that lead to boredom, frustration, and high drop-out rates.

Sounds great, doesn't it? Given all this new information, anyone who really wants to ought to be able to shape up in a matter of months. Yet, part of my job as a fitness professional is to travel all over the country, talking to and working out with women and men at all levels of the exercise field, and what I've learned is that more women than ever are feeling discouraged about getting in shape. Some of them have been doing their leg lifts and donkey kicks faithfully for a year or more without seeing much in the way of results. Others are having trouble sticking with exercise programs that, in my opinion, would make even a saint duck out and head for the nearest pizza parlor. All of them, it seems, are still trying to tone up and trim down in ways that just don't pay off very well for the amount of time and effort invested. That's why I decided to write this book.

Trading Old Ideas for New

For many years, the standard method of toning and strengthening the body was calisthenics. Despite the fact that calisthenics produced only limited results in exchange for a great deal of time and energy expended, instructors continued to teach the same old routines, or trendy variations of the same old routines, without ever really knowing why they were doing it.

We know now that there is a better way. Isotonic resistance training—that is, exercise that requires the muscles to move against resistance—has been demonstrated over and over again to be the fastest, most effective way to tone and strengthen muscles and to reshape the body. By far the most convenient form of resistance training, and the one that can be adjusted most easily to different body types and levels of conditioning, is exercise with free weights.

Free weights are ideal for home workouts because they're inexpensive and easy to store, which gives them two big advantages over the other popular form of resistance training, exercise machines. I have nothing against machines, but if you have to join a gym or a health club—and worse, get there—in order to work out on them, they allow an enormous margin for excuses and inertia to win out over good intentions. As I see it, any equipment that makes it easy for you to stick to your program is better than any equipment that makes it easy for you to cop out.

To many women, free weights still present an image problem. It's not hard to see why. When I first became interested in developing a women's free-weight program, I went looking for books on the subject. But all the books I found seemed geared only to macho men or hardcore female body builders; they were too technical as well as psychologically unappealing to women who want lean, graceful bodies instead of huge, glistening muscles or the ability to overturn cars bare-handed. For anyone not interested in body building or weight lifting as a sport, these books only perpetuated the myth of weight training as a rather bizarre obsession.

The truth is that weight training, especially as it's done in my program, is very different from either body building or weight lifting. Body builders devote themselves to building big muscles, usually for the purpose of displaying them in competition. Weight lifters work at developing the power and skill to lift very heavy weights in specialized ways. Weight training, by contrast, is nothing more or less than using weights as tools to strengthen, tone, and condition the muscles and to reshape the body into more pleasing proportions.

The big question for many women remains: will working out with free weights makes me develop big muscles, like a man? The answer is emphatically *no*. Men can build big muscles, if they work at it, because they produce an abundant supply of the male hormone testosterone, which is necessary for massive muscle growth. Women produce only small amounts of testosterone, enough to allow for adequate muscle development, but not enough to turn them into incredible hulks. The female body builders you see in magazines have to spend a great deal of time lifting heavy weights to develop the sharply-delineated muscles needed for competition. In order to get big, defined muscles, women must either have unusual genetic capability for it, or they must resort to taking steroids.

Although you won't build big muscles with the Winning Workout program, the precise effects of your workouts will depend, to some extent, on your body type. If you are an endomorph, full of curves with very little visible muscle tone, you will see improvement in your overall shape and you'll trim down heavy areas without having to worry about building muscle bulk. If you are a mesomorph with a basically muscular body that may have turned flabby from lack of exercise—particularly around your waist, hips, and thighs—you'll see a dramatic increase in muscle tone, more muscle definition, and a noticeably leaner, firmer look, especially in your problem areas. And if you are an ectomorph, one of those women who tend to look fragile and willowy even though they are often out of shape, you'll find it fairly easy to trade sagging, unhealthy-looking flesh for a better-conditioned, better-proportioned body that's lean and strong but still very graceful and feminine.

The Total Fitness Program

Keep in mind that while free weights are the basis of the Winning Workout program, they're by no means the whole of it. One of the things we've learned in the last decade or so of working with athletes and exercise buffs is that *total* fitness involves three components: strength, cardiovascular endurance, and flexibility. It makes no sense to concentrate on one of these at the expense of the others. You've probably seen runners who can do five or ten miles a day without even seeming to be out of breath, but who still have trouble reaching over their potbellies to touch their toes— or weight lifters who can't run a block without gasping for breath.

Total fitness requires balancing the three elements of fitness so that you look good, perform well, and build up your body's defenses against injury and illness. Achieving that balance doesn't have to take a lot of time, but it does require the right combination of activities. That's why I've included a chapter on a new kind of aerobic workout that is safe for virtually anyone healthy enough to exercise (but do check with your doctor before beginning this, or *any* exercise program). In Chapter 9 I'll show you how and when to stretch properly in order to reach your own maximum level of flexibility. The aerobics and stretching sections aren't just thrown in for good measure; they're an essential part of your 12-week Winning Workout program. You can do all three components of the program—aerobic workouts, free weight training, and stretching—and still keep your exercise sessions to about one hour a day, three days a week.

If part of your goal is to lose pounds as well as lose inches and to tone up what's already there, then I'd strongly advise you to spend a little extra time on your aerobic workouts. Weight training will make you look thinner by replacing fat tissue with lean muscle mass (which weighs more but takes up much less room than fat tissue) and by reshaping problem areas. But aerobics are still your best bet for dropping pounds. Provided you're in good enough condition, try to work up to 30 or 40 minutes of non-impact aerobics (you'll find out about these in Chapter 4). Added to your free-weight workouts, this will create a powerful trim-down/tone-up combination guaranteed to bring about dramatic changes in your appearance over the next 12 weeks.

What It's All About

Whether you stick to the basic program, add extra aerobics, or spend a few more minutes on the stretch section at the end of your workouts, you're going to look and feel much better after doing this program. There's really nothing magical about it: the exercises are effective, and 12 weeks is about the length of time it takes for a good program to begin to bring about visible results. The *magic* that I'm hoping will have taken hold of you by the end of the program is something more than finally liking the way you look in a swimsuit. I can't emphasize enough that the real purpose of working out is not to develop your body, but to develop your *self*—your mind, your emotions, and your relationship to the world and to the people in it.

The reason I got into fitness wasn't to shape up my mind; it was to shape up my life. At the time, I had just lost both my parents, and I was feeling totally lost and depressed. Finally, I turned to running. Although I practically had to be dragged around the track my first time out, I soon found that running lifted my spirits, focused me, and helped me clear out the cobwebs. I came back from each run positively glowing, and this eventually helped me find some of the answers I was looking for. Later, because of that experience, I became interested in other forms of exercise and ultimately chose the exercise field as a profession.

Most people don't start a fitness program because they've just had a personal tragedy, but I've worked with enough beginners to know that whatever their reasons for starting to exercise, the mental uplift they get from a fitness program always turns out to be one of their greatest rewards. The better a beginner's physical condition becomes, the more confident she feels in other areas. With weight training, that process reinforces itself: being able to *see* yourself becoming leaner and stronger has the effect of making you feel inwardly stronger. A chain reaction sets in: as you develop strength and endurance, you find that you're able to do things by yourself that you used to depend on other people to help you with, or to do for you. As a result, you feel more in charge of your life. At that point, strength is no longer the ability to lift some heavy object, but a sense of assurance that you can cope with any little crises—and maybe even some of the big ones—that come your way.

It's important to look at the whole picture. Even within the exercise field, a lot of women have fallen into the trap of thinking that being fit means having thin thighs. Sure, you can tone up your thighs, but if you don't understand that your thigh is part of your leg, and your leg is part of a physical and mental system, and *that* system is part of a whole social system, then you're missing out on an awful lot. After all, people are social animals, and if you can involve your family and friends in activities that are fun, healthy, and that build both strength and camaraderie, then I think you're getting the best of both worlds.

One of the most encouraging things I've seen in traveling around the country is the number of people—especially women—who are coming together through fitness. Women are beginning to do things most of them wouldn't have dreamed of doing ten or twenty years ago—organizing basketball and volleyball leagues, going hiking with their families—being participants instead of spectators. I think it's great that when a date calls up, a woman can just as easily go bicycling or rock climbing as go to the movies. For married women, being fit can mean not staying home while your husband goes golfing, and joining in when the rest of your family plays softball on the lawn.

Being fit means being ready, mentally and physically, to participate in life. If we've learned anything over the last few years, our daughters will get a better jump on the game: maybe they'll grow up feeling more at ease with their bodies, and maybe, just maybe, they won't have to spend their whole lives worrying about their weight. If we can start to get in shape as a group, as a team, as a family, and as a country, maybe we can begin to have a stronger, healthier America.

CHAPTER ONE

In Tune

There are two ways to approach an exercise program. The first is merely to go through the motions, mechanically performing leg lifts while you plan your dinner menu and pray the workout will soon be over. The second is to tune into yourself, becoming sensitive to your body's responses and aware of the constant interplay of muscle and movement. With enough patience and consistent effort, the first approach will, eventually, help you trim your thighs and flatten your stomach—that is, if you don't die of boredom before the routine has a chance to work. But I know I could never stick to this kind of program, and I don't see why you should—especially given the fact that one movement performed with true body awareness is as effective as twenty mindless repetitions.

The real rewards of getting in tune with your body go far beyond cosmetic results. To me, exercising without physical awareness seems a little like making love while wearing ski clothes: sure, you can probably maneuver it, but you're certainly going to miss out on the subtleties, if not the purpose of the whole experience. This analogy isn't as far-fetched as it may sound, because I'm suggesting that you can develop an *intimate relationship* with your own body through a thoughtful exercise program. That means having the same kind of caring, trusting, and forgiving feelings towards yourself that you have toward the people you love. It means nurturing your best qualities and refusing to get hung up on your imperfections, so that you can get on with life with good grace and a spirit of adventure. And if this sounds like some pop psychologist's vague admonition to "get in touch with yourself," it's anything but; working out and getting fit *is* a down-to-earth, nuts-and-bolts way to get in touch with yourself. It's learning by doing instead of just wishing.

In this chapter, I'm going to suggest some mental and physical exercises that will show you what it's like to be in tune with yourself. Except for the Mirror Checklist, these exercises can be done a little at a time, whenever you have a few minutes of peace and quiet. None of them should feel like work; they're meant only to teach you to relax at will, to cope with stress, to understand your body's signals, and to enjoy your workouts. Do approach them with patience, however. Remember that you're learning valuable new skills, and learning any skill is a process, not an overnight transformation.

Making a Mirror Checklist

Presumably, you're starting this exercise program because you want to make certain changes in the way you look. In order to make changes effectively, you need a clear idea of where you're starting *from*. The purpose of making the Mirror Checklist is to give you, perhaps for the first time in your life, a realistic view of your body as it is—not as you secretly hope or fear it is—so that you can set specific goals for yourself and make tangible improvements.

Give yourself half an hour or so of private time. Pluck up your courage, get undressed, and stand in front of a full-length mirror. Have the Mirror Checklist (p. 13), the Self-Portrait Page (p. 14), and a pencil ready because, believe it or not, you're going to be taking notes. Take an overall look at your body. The important thing to remember at this point is *not to criticize!* If you hear any nagging, reproachful mental voices making insulting comments about your hips or bustline, just tell them calmly and firmly to shut up; this exercise is about getting to know your body, not about judging it.

Turn to the Mirror Checklist and note the date, and your weight and height. With your tape measure, take your measurements for A through K, and record them in the appropriate spaces. You can take these measurements each week through the 12-week program to check your progress.

Next, look at your body structure and see if you can determine your body type. Make sure, as you proceed, that you check yourself out thoroughly from the front, side, and back views—very few of us ever really look at ourselves from behind.

Are you mainly soft and rounded, full of voluptuous curves and covered by a layer of body fat that appears to be distributed more or less evenly over your entire body? If you fit this description, you're probably an *endomorph*, and, as I pointed out in the Introduction, you're going to be able to whittle down the too-fleshy areas of your body without developing much visible muscle. Take a closer look at your proportions. Do some parts of your body seem much larger in relation to others? Endomorphs often collect fat around their abdomen, hips, and thighs, making them appear bottom-heavy. If this is true for you, you're going to want to work at trimming fat below the waist while you develop more muscle above the waist, to give your body a more balanced appearance.

You may, however, be more of a *mesomorph*—thicker-boned and generally more athletic-looking, (even if you happen to be out of shape right now). Look closely at your proportions again. Does anything seem out of balance? If so, is it because of fat deposits, muscle development, or bone structure? One of the things you need to determine in this exercise is precisely what can and what can't be changed about your body. We can do something about rearranging fat and muscle, but obviously, we can't do much about the bone structure you were born with.

Ectomorphs, the thin, fragile, "waif" types I mentioned in the Introduction, can be overweight or underweight, but they all tend to have an angular look and few discernible muscles. Often ectomorphs need to firm up flesh that sags due to lack of muscle tone, and build up cetain areas that look unattractively flat or "caved in."

Keep in mind, as you evaluate your body structure, that no two bodies are exactly alike, and yours probably combines elements of more than one body type. Just try to get the clearest possible picture of your basic bone structure and of the way fat and muscle are distributed over your body. Then take a minute to write down what you've learned about your body type on the Self-Portrait Page.

Now check your mirror image again to see how you carry yourself. Once again, make sure you evaluate your front, side, and back views equally. Look at your spine: is it relatively straight, or are you swaybacked? If the latter is true, you'll probably also notice when you turn to the side that your abdomen is protruding. Do you carry most of your weight over your heels, or forward over the balls of your feet? Are your shoulders and chest hunched forward, pulled back, or do you hold your chest high with your shoulders lowered and relaxed? Do your shoulder blades jut out in back when you stand straight?

The picture you're getting as you evaluate your posture and alignment will tell you a great deal about how to correct certain body problems, which often are more a matter of poor carriage than of excess fat. It will also give you some valuable insights into the way you *feel* about your body, and remind you that the caved-in chest, the pelvis left to trail unassertively behind, and the defeated slump of shoulders are what you're projecting to the rest of the world—in other words, what you're asking others to feel about you, too. Again, once you've finished your evaluation, make a note of what you've discovered about your posture and alignment.

The next step is to make a more detailed observation of your body, from your toes up. Think of yourself as an artist making a study for a portrait, and try to gather as much information as possible. Observe the length, width, and overall shape of your feet; look at the way your toes are formed, the shape and condition of your toenails, and the texture of

Mirror Checklist

This chart will give you a written record of the progress you achieve while performing your Winning Workout program.

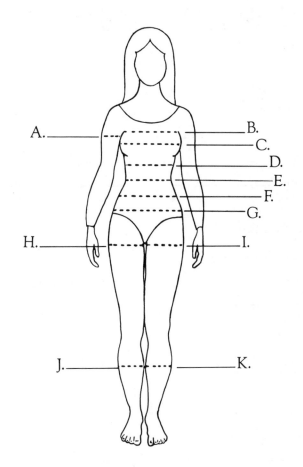

DATE													
Weight													
Height													
A. Upper arm													
B. Upper chest													
C. Bustline													
D. Midriff													
E. Waistline													
F. Upper hips													
G. Hips													
H. Right thigh													
I. Left thigh													
J. Right calf													
K. Left calf													

Self-Portrait Page

My body type:

endomorph_____

mesomorph_____

ectomorph_____

Notes on my body type and bone structure:

_____

_____

_____

_____

My bone structure:

small_____

medium_____

large_____

_____

_____

_____

My posture and alignment:

spine:_____

shoulders:_____

chest:_____

abdomen:_____

Overall Observations:

_____

_____

_____

_____

Features I like:

_____

_____

_____

_____

_____

_____

_____

Features I'll learn to accept:

_____

_____

_____

_____

_____

_____

_____

Features I can change:

_____

_____

_____

_____

_____

_____

_____

the skin around them. As you review each part of your body, be equally precise and dispassionate. The clearer and more detailed the picture you form, the easier it will be for you to deal with what you see, and to begin to let go of the emotional baggage that keeps most of us from ever effecting the changes we dream of making.

Finally, you're ready for what is, in a way, the moment of truth in the mirror exercise. This time, I want you to scan your body again and jot down what you like and what you don't like. Then determine which features that you *don't* like can be changed—and which ones cannot. By now, you should be able to view your imperfections without panic or self-loathing. You should be in a position to make a realistic assessment of what you can do to improve your looks, and to begin to accept those things about yourself that are hereditary and unchangeable. If you think of how other members of your immediate family were built, you'll realize that some of your features are things you were born with and may as well learn to like, because you'll be living with them for the rest of your life. The more gracefully you can accept the things you can't change, the easier it will be to get on with the task of changing those you can.

Make a note of your decisions, listing the features you like in the first column, those you feel you can't do anything about in the second column, and in the third column, those that require action. Read over your list to determine how you are going to deal with your "can change" entries. Many of them will call for improvement through exercise, but others may be a matter of paying more attention to grooming, reevaluating some of your attitudes, or simply learning how to focus attention on your best features and downplay your flaws.

How ever your list shapes up, you should congratulate yourself. Do you know how many people go through life without ever knowing what they really look like? You've just made more headway than you realize.

Knowing Your Way Around

Since your body is where you live, you'll naturally feel more confident in it if you know a little about its geography. I'm not going to burden you with a lot of technical information, but you might want to familiarize yourself with the names and functions of some of the muscle groups we'll be working with so that when I refer to them later, you won't feel that you're reading a foreign language. Check the accompanying diagrams to get a more complete idea of your body's muscular layout.

Muscle Groups — Front View

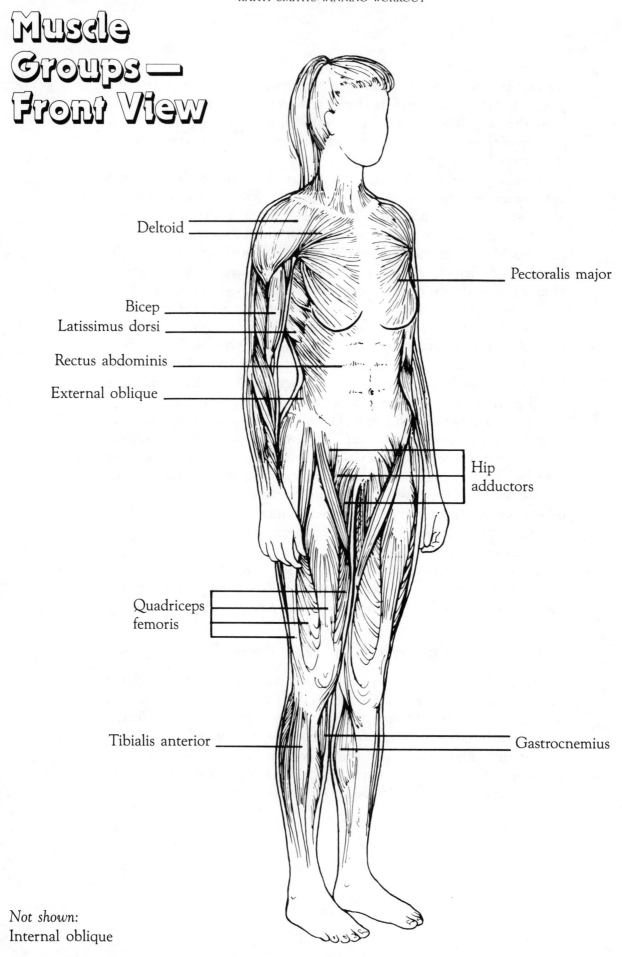

Deltoid

Pectoralis major

Bicep

Latissimus dorsi

Rectus abdominis

External oblique

Hip adductors

Quadriceps femoris

Tibialis anterior

Gastrocnemius

Not shown:
Internal oblique

Muscle Groups — Rear View

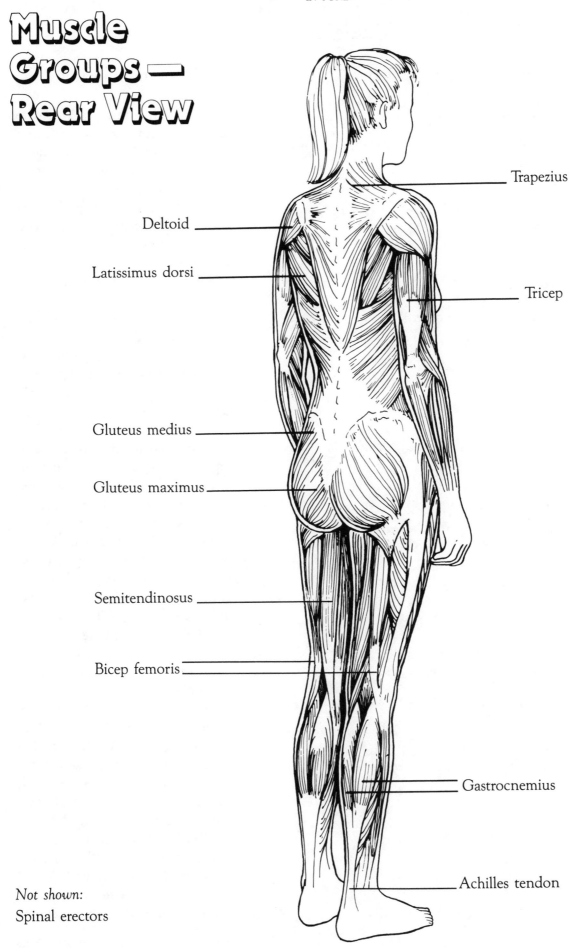

Trapezius

Deltoid

Latissimus dorsi

Tricep

Gluteus medius

Gluteus maximus

Semitendinosus

Bicep femoris

Gastrocnemius

Achilles tendon

Not shown:
Spinal erectors

Muscle Groups

Anatomical Name	Slang Term	Location and Function
Trapezius	traps	The trapezius muscles originate along your spine and extend in a triangle over your shoulders, upper back, and the back of your neck. They enable you to shrug your shoulders and pull them back, and to keep your head erect. Strengthening your trapezius muscles can help correct rounded shoulders and a jutting chin.
Deltoids	delts	The deltoids are the shoulder muscles located at the tops of your arms, outside your trapezius muscles. They help you lift your arms. These muscles tend to be poorly developed, especially in women.
Latissimus dorsi	lats	The "lats" cover the broadest area of your back, spreading out from either side of your spine, just below your waist, to the undersides of your arms. They allow you to move and twist your back, and help you pull your arms in and your shoulders down. When flab collects around untoned "lats," you get the tops of "love handles" and below-the-bra bulges.
Pectoralis major	pecs	The pectoral muscles extend over your chest in two sections: the upper and lower "pecs." Proper development of both groups gives you a high, proud chest and a lifted bustline, and is essential for proper breathing. A sunken, caved-in chest, the result of weak "pecs" and poor posture, leads to shallow breathing and the chronic fatigue that often afflicts people who sit slumped over desks all day. Luckily, these muscles respond very readily to resistance exercises.

Anatomical Name	Slang Term	Location and Function
Biceps		The biceps are the front of your upper arms, and they're what help you lift the groceries—or, if you're like most women, what *don't* help you lift the groceries. Like the "pecs," these can be strengthened quickly with free weights.
Triceps		The triceps are at the backs of your upper arms. They allow you to lower your arms once you've lifted them, and to pull your arms back. Most women have difficulty keeping this area well-toned. The result is that as we get older, we tend to develop loose, flabby tissue on the backs of our upper arms. These muscles are extremely difficult to tone, except through resistance exercises.
Spinal erectors		Extending up either side of your spinal column, the spinal erectors form the support columns for your back, and help your pelvis bear the pressure of your body weight. They must be trained carefully, since they lack the bony support provided for other muscles. However, for most people, trouble comes not from over-exercising the spinal erectors, but from under-exercising the abdominals, which shortens the spinal erectors and sways the back, leading to lower back pain.
Gluteals	glutes	There are three groups of gluteals: the gluteus maximus, which forms the large, globular part of your buttocks; the gluteus medius, which runs from your hipbones to the tops of your thighbones and contours your hips; and the gluteus minimus, which works

Anatomical Name	Slang Term	Location and Function
(Gluteals, cont'd.)		with the gluteus medius to raise your legs to the sides. The "glutes," as you probably already know, can be real trouble zones, since they tend to collect fatty deposits more readily than any other muscle group.
Rectus abdominis	abs	The all-important abdominals, running up the center of the torso, are crucial to your posture, appearance, and overall health. They need to be exercised very regularly, since they deteriorate faster than any other muscle group in your body.
Obliques, internal and external		Located on either side of the rectus abdominus, the obliques help the "abs" maintain correct alignment of the back and pelvis. Often neglected, they need to be strengthened and toned because they have an important supportive role and because a thick waistline and "love handles" can develop when they are allowed to deteriorate.
Quadriceps femoris	quads	The quadriceps are a set of four muscles that run down the front of your thighs to your knees. Their job is to extend your legs and to protect your knee joints. Since women's hips are set at a wider angle to the knees than men's, strong quadriceps are doubly important to help women avoid knee injuries. Pouchy, sagging flesh just over your kneecaps is a sure sign that your "quads" need work.
Semitendinosus and Bicep femoris	hamstrings	The hamstrings are the quadriceps' opposites, running up and down the backs of your thighs. They allow you to bend your

Anatomical Name	Slang Term	Location and Function
(Hamstrings, contd.)		knees, rotate your legs, and extend your legs backward. To insure safe, balanced movement, your hamstrings and your quads must be stretched and strengthened equally. Many activities, such as running, tend to develop one group at the expense of the other.
Hip adductors		The muscles of the insides of your thighs, these muscles run from your groin to various points along your thigh bones, and act to pull your knees together. It's extremely difficult to tone these muscles unless you do some form of resistance exercise.
Gastrocnemius	gastroc	The major calf muscles, the "gastrocs" are divided into two sections, one on the outside of your calf and one on the inside. These muscles tend to be fairly strong but rather inflexible, since we keep them contracted so much of the time. It's important to warm them up thoroughly and stretch them out frequently when you exercise, in order to avoid injuring them.
Tibialis anterior	shins	Commonly known as the shins, these muscles allow you to flex your feet. They're rarely well-developed in non-athletes, but they should be strengthened in order to balance the hard-working "gastrocs" on the other side of the calves.

Working with Your Natural Cycles

It's still surprising to me to realize how out of touch I used to be with my own natural cycles. For years I was unconscious of when I was about to get my periods, and unwilling to admit that they had any real effect on me. Because I've always been athletic, menstruation never was as much of a problem for me as it is for many women, but I used to act as if it simply didn't exist.

Then I began working with a fitness trainer who insisted that I keep a training record, jotting down not only what comprised my workouts each day, but also how I felt during them. The result was a revelation. Over a period of weeks, then months, I began to see that my performance, my energy level, my emotional state, and even my susceptibility to illness, all formed definite patterns that did, in fact, correspond to my menstrual cycles, and to even subtler circadian rhythms.

Understanding that there was a *reason* for the variations in my performance allowed me to relax and work with the changes, instead of feeling confused and discouraged. It was as if a light had been turned on in my mind, and I began to have a greater understanding and awareness of myself as a whole, interconnected system. This, in turn, made me aware of the ways in which a whole spectrum of external factors—the foods I'd eaten, the amount of sleep I'd had, the ups and downs in my career and personal life—all affected my performance. The clearer the correlation between these outside influences and my performance became, the more motivated—and the better-equipped—I was to modify certain aspects of my lifestyle so that I could feel as good as possible. All along, my body had been sending me coded signals. Now that I'd cracked the code, I had a constant, reassuring sense of being tuned in to my own physiological needs and of being able to do something about them.

My experience certainly wasn't unique. Many athletes have discovered that keeping a training diary is an enormous help, both in motivating them to stick to their training programs, and in teaching them how to maximize their potential. For anyone about to start the Winning Workout program, keeping a diary will be an invaluable tool. For one thing, it's a great way to tune into and understand your body as a *system*, connected with and responsive to a host of internal and external factors. For another, when you're just beginning an exercise program, knowing how to interpret a few "off" days or an apparently unwarranted weight gain as part of a natural cycle, rather than proof that you or your techniques have failed, can mean the difference between sticking with the program until you can claim your rewards, or giving up before you reach the finish line.

Your training diary doesn't have to be anything elaborate—I keep mine right on my daily calendar. Just jot down the time of day you exercised, what your workout consisted of, how you felt, and any unusual circumstances that may have affected your performance. If you're trying to lose weight, you should certainly add a note about what you ate during the day as well. The whole process needn't take more than a couple of minutes.

Once you've established the habit of keeping your diary, make sure you review it every week or two. You'll be amazed at how much you can learn about yourself in a very short time.

Learning to Let Go

Until now, I've been asking you to get to know yourself from the outside. Now I'd like you to start feeling comfortable with yourself on the *inside*, too. Progressive Relaxation is a technique that can help you feel more at ease with yourself and more in control of your actions, can increase your physical awareness, and can help you tap into your hidden reserves of energy. Relaxing should be a simple process, but most of us are so accustomed to high levels of stress and muscle tension in our daily lives that simply letting go can seem virtually impossible. Give yourself time to let the Progressive Relaxation technique sink in. No one masters it on the first try, or on the second. It's a process that demands a little patience, a little faith, and lots of practice, but if you give it just ten minutes a day, I promise you that you'll soon be able to relax your body and refresh your mind at will, whenever you feel you need a break from stress. Here's how it works:

Sit or lie in a comfortable position, with your feet uncrossed and your hands resting easily at your sides. Begin by focusing on your breathing. Breathe deeply and naturally, allowing your abdomen to expand as you inhale and contract as you exhale. If you're not sure you're breathing correctly, lie down and put both hands on your abdomen. When you inhale, your hands should rise; when you exhale, they should fall as your abdomen sinks. As you continue to breathe deeply and rhythmically, become aware of the sensation of air flowing in and out of your body. Each time you exhale, think of letting go of tension; each time you inhale, think of taking in fresh energy. Don't try to control your breath, just remain aware of it.

Now focus your attention on your feet and try to relax the muscles in them, one by one. Imagine that your feet are very heavy and warm. Feel them become more and more relaxed.

Work your way slowly up your body, focusing carefully on your ankles, your calves, your thighs, your pelvis, your abdomen, your chest, your arms, all the way out to your fingers, and then up to your face. Pay particular attention to areas where you are habitually tense: for instance, your shoulders, neck, and jaw. Spend a little extra time on these areas and see if you can imagine each of them becoming loose, smooth, and totally relaxed. Don't rush. This is a mini-vacation from everyday anxieties and pressures, so try to enjoy it.

Once you've worked your way up through your whole body, go back and scan each muscle group again, searching for areas of residual tension. Is there any tightness left in your scalp? Roll your neck around very gently to make sure you've really loosened *those* muscles. Check the subtle hiding places of tension, like the area where little lines form around your eyes. Let each of these places relax, one by one. Feel that your whole body is totally relaxed and comfortable, and that your mind is quiet.

When you're ready to come back to your normal, alert state, just take three deep breaths and open your eyes. Once you've mastered the art of Progressive Relaxation, you'll feel, at this moment, as if you'd just come back from a weekend in the country.

Visualization

I firmly believe that you can only be as good as you can imagine yourself being. You'll never be president of your own company if you can't imagine yourself as more than a messenger; you'll never be good at sports if you can only imagine yourself being clumsy; you'll never be thin if you can't see yourself as anything but fat. You have to be able to dream what you want in order to be it.

As it happens, this isn't just my personal belief. The Soviet Union's top athletes have long made visualization—the technique of seeing yourself performing an action exactly as you would like to perform it—an integral part of their training programs. Over the past few years, American trainers have begun to use visualization with equal success. This technique can work for you, too. Visualization is most effective when mind and body are deeply relaxed, as they are in the last phase of Progressive Relaxation. To give it a try, go through your Progressive Relaxation sequence until you feel deeply relaxed. Then, with your eyes closed, picture a setting, either a real place you've seen or an imaginary landscape, that represents your idea of perfect tranquility. For you this might be a tropical beach with palm trees swaying in the breeze; or it could be a flowery meadow or a grassy hillside. Whatever you imagine, try to see it as clearly and in as much detail as possible. Let the picture relax you even more deeply.

After a while, you should feel as if you are floating peacefully somewhere between sleep and wakefulness. When you reach this point, or at least a very calm state in which your mind floats free, change your mental image and picture yourself as you would like to look. You might want to imagine yourself standing in front of a mirror, or walking down the street; but try to see yourself in as much detail as possible. See the areas of your body that you most want to change, and imagine them lean and well-toned. Look at your mental picture from all sides; get the overall effect. *Dream* yourself in your ideal image. Stay with the image for a while before you let it float away.

By practicing this type of visualization often, you'll build the image of your ideal body into your mental framework. As you become more and more familiar with your ideal body image and make it a part of you, you will learn to do what competitive athletes have learned to do: rehearse for success.

Concentration

Concentration is a key factor in doing anything well, but it plays an especially vital role in working with free weights. By focusing your attention on contracting only the muscles you are working on in a given exercise, you can work those muscles very specifically and intensely, without letting other parts of the body lessen the effects by "helping." Maintaining your concentration throughout each full set of repetitions will produce dramatic results and will make your workouts more interesting.

Luckily, the concentration that's needed for a free-weight workout is considerably easier to develop than that needed for tennis, for example, in which your mind must remain alert to many different factors at once, from your opponent's shots to the wind and the surface of the court. Still, if you're used to daydreaming in exercise class while your instructor counts off repetitions, learning to maintain concentration and body awareness may take practice.

One of the best concentration-builders I've ever found is yoga. Studying yoga with Bikram at the Yoga College of India taught me how to focus intently on one action at a time while remaining aware of my body's responses and screening out all distractions. The three exercises I demonstrate here are adapted from my yoga training. Try them and you'll get an immediate sense of what focused body awareness is all about; practice them until you can do them easily, and you'll have a good grasp of the fine art of concentration.

1. The Imaginary Chair

STEP A

Stand with feet shoulder-width apart, arms extended forward at shoulder level. Rise onto your toes and hold this position for five seconds.

STEP B

Now bend your knees, keeping your back straight and your chest lifted, and lower yourself to a sitting position. Focus on a point in front of you and tune into your body cues. Hold the position for 30 seconds.

THE INNER GAME

As you begin this exercise, find a point in front of you at eye level (it helps to find a real point; for example, a scratch on the wall). Focus on that point and block out the rest of your surroundings.

Once you've risen to your toes, go through a mental body check: Are your hands flat and relaxed? Shoulders down? Elbows and back straight? Stomach and buttocks tight? Are you breathing easily and normally, or holding your breath?

As you sit in the Imaginary Chair, keep focusing on the point in front of you while you tune into body cues: notice whether your ankles are wobbly, and if they are, try to stabilize them. If you start to feel a burning sensation in your thighs, remain aware of it and notice that if you squeeze your inner thighs a bit, the burning will lessen.

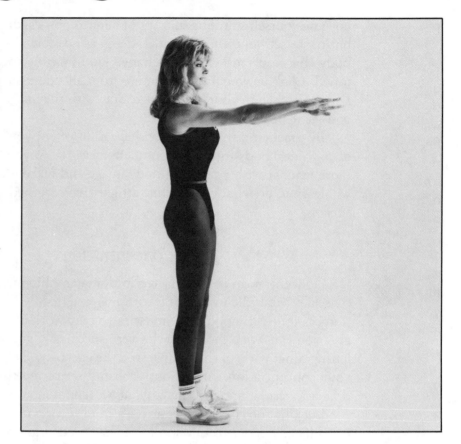

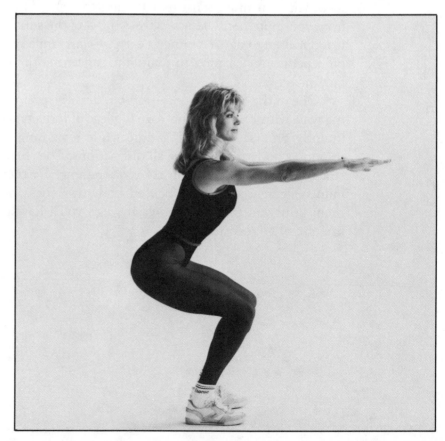

2. Standing Head-to-Knee

BEGINNER'S POSITION

Stand on your left leg with your knee straight and your quadricep muscle pulled up tight. Bring your right knee toward your chest. Interlock your fingers under the ball of your right foot. Beginners should try to hold this position for 30 seconds, then repeat the exercise on their left leg.

ADVANCED POSITION

If you're more advanced, extend your right leg in front of you until the knee is straight, and bring your head down to your knee. Hold the position for 30 seconds, then repeat on your left leg.

THE INNER GAME

If you are a beginner, focus on a spot on the floor about three feet in front of you and maintain that focus while you hold the position. If you're more advanced, focus on a spot right next to the inside of your standing foot. In both positions, concentrate on keeping your standing leg absolutely straight and stable, like a pillar of marble.

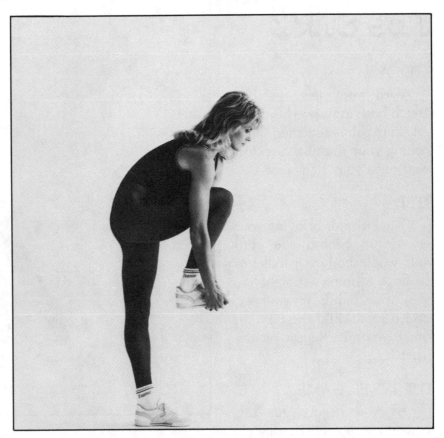

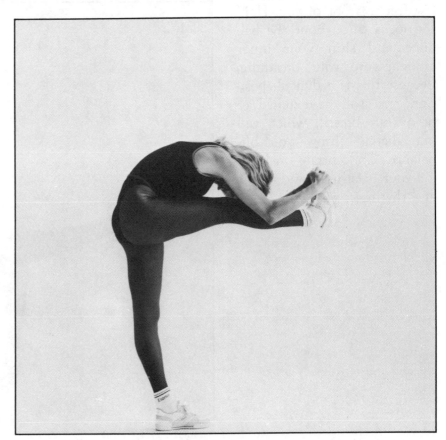

3.
The Stick

STEP A

With your feet together, stretch both arms overhead and put your palms together, interlocking your thumbs. Step forward onto your right foot.

STEP B

Tilt forward, bringing your left leg up behind you until your whole body is parallel to the floor, forming a straight line from your hands to your extended foot. Hold the position for 30 seconds. Repeat on the other leg.

THE INNER GAME

As you begin your tilt, focus on a spot on the floor a few feet in front of you. Hold the focus throughout the balance and shift your inner awareness to your breathing. Because this is a difficult position, you will be tempted to hold your breath, which will immediately throw you off-balance. Concentrate on keeping your breathing easy, steady, and rhythmic.

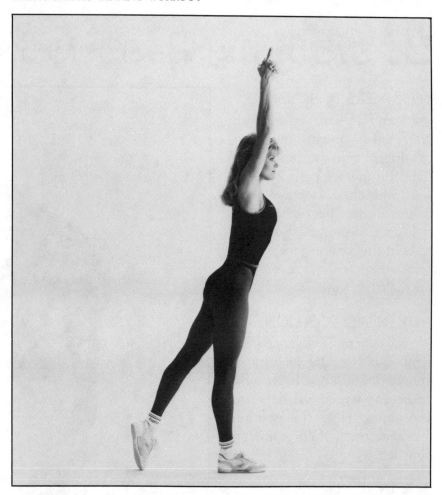

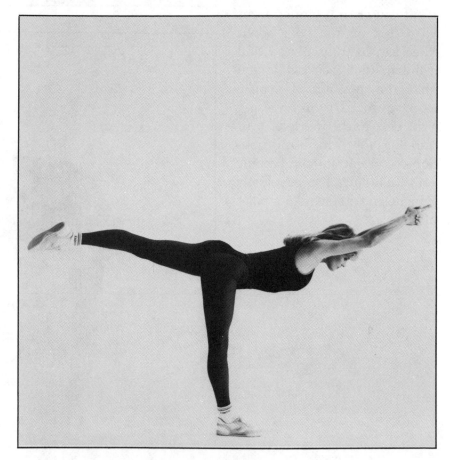

Russell Clark's 8-Step Tune-up

Russell Clark is a friend of mine who is a terrific jazz dancer and teacher. In his Los Angeles dance classes, he teaches all levels of students and puts great emphasis on body awareness as a key to fluid, sensuous movement. To prepare his students for tricky dance combinations, he takes them through a tune-up exercise that helps them get in touch with their bodies before they start to move. This eight-step routine combines mind and muscle to wake up the body instantly. You can use it anywhere, anytime, to gear up for your workout or whenever you feel the need to get body and soul together quickly.

This routine is like an add-on game: you not only do each step in sequence, but you must also continue to do all of the preceding steps as you add each new one.

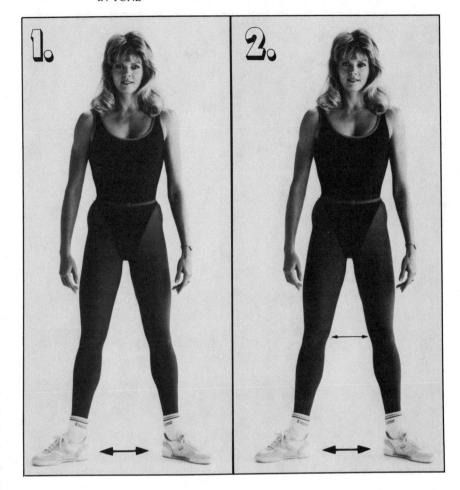

1. Stand with your legs apart and your feet turned out slightly. Without actually moving your feet, pull your heels together, as if you were on roller skates.

2. Pull your knees together without actually moving them.

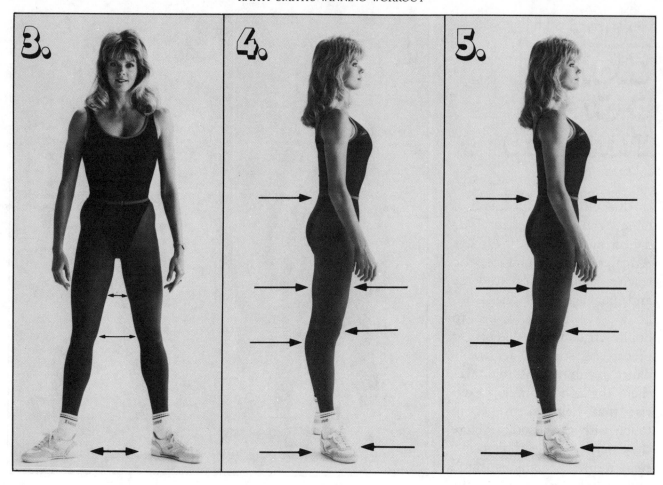

3. Pull your thighs together without actually moving them.

4. Tighten your buttocks as you press your tailbone straight down (don't tuck it under, though) and lengthen your spine.

5. Pull your navel towards your spine.

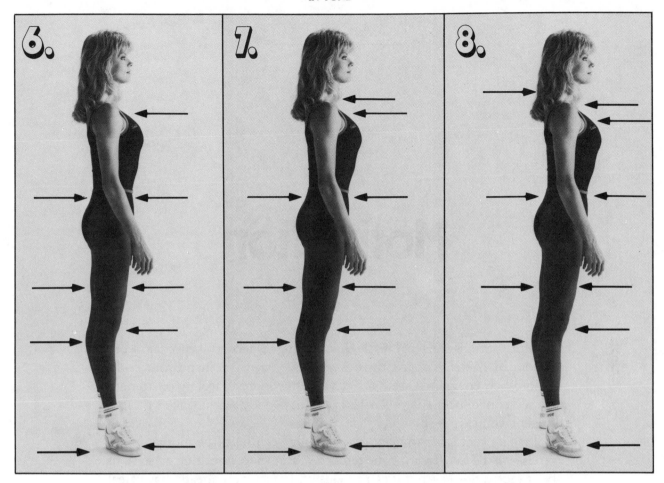

6. Lift your chest as if you were being pulled upward by a string attached to your sternum.

7. Lower your shoulders.

8. Lengthen your neck, as though another string were pulling you up by the crown of your head.

CHAPTER TWO

Motivation

Motivation is the real muscle that is going to make this program work for you. In 12 weeks, using these workouts, you will reshape your body, tap into new energy reserves, and develop a wonderful feeling of strength and self-confidence. All you have to do, as Woody Allen once said in a different context, is show up.

I realize that for many people, especially beginners, the motivation to exercise can be here today, gone tomorrow. But there's nothing mysterious about motivation, even if it can be elusive. In fact, you already have great stores of motivation working for you. You're motivated to get out of bed in the morning, to go to work, to buy new clothes, and to eat dinner. Motivation is what makes things happen in your life. Now it's going to make things happen in your body. All we need to do is to channel your existing drive into making you lean, strong, and healthy.

There are very specific factors, we've discovered, that can help people stick to exercise. Many of these have already been built into the Winning Workout program. You won't have to think about them to feel their effects; they'll simply make these routines easier to stick to than those you may have tried in the past. I'll be telling you about some others in this chapter. Think of them as tricks of the trade: if you learn to use them, they'll keep your morale high and your enthusiasm alive until you can claim the rewards of your efforts.

First, I want you to understand that motivation—the kind of motivation we'll be using for the next 12 weeks—isn't will power, it's *want* power. I believe that the more you want something, the more you're willing to do to get it, without having to punish yourself or feel deprived. A strong desire will pull you forward like a magnet, making it easier to cope with the obstacles and interruptions that will inevitably crop up along the way. That's why, as sports psychologists have discovered, setting definite goals is the first step in assuring success.

Setting Realistic Goals

Goals must fit three criteria in order to work: they must be clear, they must be challenging, and they must be attainable. Think back to your Mirror Checklist. Which of the things on your "can change" list would you most like to accomplish in the next 12 weeks? Remember that your goals must be attainable. Realistically, you can't expect to lose 100 pounds and 14 inches off your hips in three months but you *might* decide to lose 15 pounds and three inches. You might decide to build your upper body so that it's in proportion to your lower half. Or you could decide to develop enough strength to carry both your child and your groceries without feeling exhausted. Or you may choose to get rid of cottage-cheese thighs and develop a more beautiful line to your legs.

Once you've decided on your goals, write them down. They'll come in handy the next time you're tempted to spend a rainy Sunday in bed eating chocolates.

At this point you don't have to be concerned about making your goals challenging. For one thing, challenge is already structured into your program, and for another, I don't know of anyone who ever set out on an exercise program with a goal of losing only $\frac{1}{16}$ of an inch from her waist!

You are, however, going to need two kinds of goals: long-term and short-term. Long-term goals are the ones we've just been considering, and they're all about results. Short-term goals, on the other hand, concern the day-to-day process involved in achieving those results. The principle behind short-term goals is that success breeds success. Experiencing lots of small victories teaches you to be a winner in the long run. Here again, you're already ahead of the game, because many short-term goals have been built into your program.

Getting through a given number of repetitions of a certain exercise on a particular day is an example of a short-term goal. These goals will become progressively more challenging as you proceed through the program. But you can make your workouts more fun and add to your sense of accomplishment by coming up with your own personal short-term goals for each session. For example, one day you might try to make all your movements look smoother and more accomplished. At the next session, you might work to keep your breathing easy and rhythmic, even during the toughest moves. Once you get used to working with free weights, the opportunities for small victories will crop up naturally. All you have to do is accept the challenge, and each workout will become more absorbing than the last.

One more thing: don't confuse long-term and short-term goals. Jumping on the scales every day, or even every week, to see how you're doing is simply counter-productive. Remember, too, that muscle weighs more than fat and that your weight is bound to fluctuate with your natural cycles. Give your program a chance to work, and learn to depend on your own eyes and feelings to measure how well your efforts are paying off.

Making a Commitment

Once you've defined your goals, your next step is to make a commitment to achieving them. This simply means accepting the responsibility for making what you *want* to happen, happen. I can promise you that at some time during the next 12 weeks, people or events will threaten to distract you from your purpose and interfere with your exercise schedule. It's important for you to realize that these external factors can't make you fail; only *you* can let yourself fail, just as only *you* can make yourself succeed.

Athletes use a training concept called *adaptability*, which, for our purposes, can be defined as adapting to circumstances to make them work for, not against, your success. For example, a runner with an injured knee may turn to swimming to keep in shape until she can return to her running routine. In the process, she may develop a new kind of strength that will utimately make her a better athlete.

We can all use the principle of adaptability on an everyday level. You don't, for instance, have to turn down all dinner invitations for the next 12 weeks because you've scheduled your workouts for 7 p.m.; you just have to rearrange your schedule to accommodate both your workouts *and* your social life. Nor do you have to abandon your workouts whenever things get too hectic at your job. You might gain something, in fact, by reorganizing your workload or by re-examining your priorities. Who knows; maybe you're being asked to carry too much of the burden, and you'll finally gather the courage to be assertive about your own needs. I can't predict all the potential obstacles to your fitness program, I can only assure you that they can all be overcome if you're willing to make a reasonable, but unshakable, commitment to your own success. Remember, blaming other people or outside events for your failures only makes you weak. Taking charge of your life gives you a sense of control—and, more importantly, allows you to trust yourself.

Planning for Success

A little planning and just a few of the right moves can make exercising so much easier that it's downright silly to neglect them:

☑ PLAN YOUR WORKOUTS

Schedule your workouts just as you would an appointment with your doctor or hairdresser, and note your appointment in your daybook or calendar. As one sports psychologist put it, one reason things often don't go according to plan is that there was no plan to begin with!

☑ LET YOUR FRIENDS IN ON YOUR PLAN

Try to engage your friends' cooperation by telling them in advance that you'll be busy at such-and-such a time, but would be delighted to get together afterward. There are all kinds of considerate ways to accommodate the needs of your family and friends, and to get them to accommodate *your* needs as well.

☑ PICK A PLEASANT PLACE TO EXERCISE

If you're planning to work out during the day, choose a place that has plenty of sunlight and fresh air. If you're an evening exerciser, look for an area of your home that is clear of furniture and well lit.

☑ LAY OUT YOUR WEIGHTS AND YOUR WORKOUT CLOTHES AHEAD OF TIME

I've often thought that the toughest part of my exercise routines is the time it takes me to change into my leotards or sweats. That's when I can be tempted into a "should-I-or-shouldn't-I" debate with myself, before the momentum of the workout gets me motivated. Make this transition as quickly and easily as you possibly can.

☑ EXERCISE TO MUSIC YOU LIKE

Don't underestimate the boost you get from good background music. A solid beat will help you keep your exercise rhythm steady, and the sheer pleasure of listening to music you like will keep you going when you start to feel fatigued. Personally, I like strong, *Chariots of Fire*-type music when I work out, but anything will do, as long as it isn't so fast that it makes your movements jerky, or so slow that it puts you to sleep.

☑ FIND AN EXERCISE BUDDY

If you can manage it, working out with a partner can make exercise a lot more fun. Just be sure that your partner is at least as committed to the program as you are, and doesn't have a schedule that is likely to conflict with your own. You don't need any bad influences in your life at *this* point.

☑ REVIEW YOUR TRAINING DIARY OFTEN

Reviewing your diary can strengthen your motivation. You training diary is also a great place to stash any fitness-related articles, pictures, clips, or quotes that inspire or interest you. When you come across them later, they'll get you fired up for exercise all over again. It's important to give yourself plenty of reminders that will keep fitness a priority in your life when a million other things are demanding your attention.

☑ USE PROGRESSIVE RELAXATION

Put yourself into a calm, relaxed state, then visualize a time in your life when you felt very good about yourself. You may have achieved something special in your work, or just formed a great personal relationship, or lost ten pounds—it doesn't matter what it was, as long as you can recall feeling good about yourself.

Try to create as detailed an image as possible of how you were at that particular time: what you looked like, and what factors may have influenced your success. Maybe you were eating very healthfully then, or getting lots of positive reinforcement from your family. Recall as many specifics as possible, so that you have a very clear image of the way you were.

Now try to recall the way you *felt* at the time. See if you can pinpoint the sensations that were associated with your success. Everyone's experience of success is different and very personal; some people associate success with feelings of competence and control, others with a sense of freedom or a lack of inhibitions. Use your visualization technique to call up *your* success feelings and practice making them part of your everyday experience.

☑ MOST IMPORTANT OF ALL: BE POSITIVE ABOUT YOURSELF AND YOUR FITNESS PROGRAM

Given half a chance, exercise is going to become one of the most rewarding, invigorating, and purely pleasurable parts of your day. When you begin to exercise regularly, your workouts will become mini-vacations from everyday stress, boredom, and anxiety. They'll be a time to refresh and refuel yourself for what's ahead.

A good workout shouldn't be work at all; it should be *play*. This is one of the rare times in your adult life when you're allowed to re-experience the physical and mental freedom you had as a child. If you convince yourself that exercise is going to be drudgery, you'll cheat yourself out of a fantastic opportunity. And if you beat yourself over the head because you slipped up and missed a workout, or ate too much, or hate the way you look in a leotard, you're missing the point. You're trying, however imperfectly, to do something good for yourself. For that you deserve praise, not punishment. The less you focus on temporary set-backs, the better your chances for ultimate success.

Stay open and enthusiastic, remember to pat yourself on the back for your efforts, and you'll soon build up such a reserve of good feelings about getting fit that just remembering how terrific you felt after your last work-out will be enough to get you psyched up for your next one.

One more word about overcoming that old demon, inertia: I've talked to a lot of sedentary, out-of-shape people over the last few years, and if there's one thing they all seem to have in common, it's that they all spend hours worrying that they don't exercise, but don't spend any time doing anything about it. Remember the scientific rule: "A body in motion tends to stay in motion; a body at rest tends to stay at rest." The next time you find yourself conducting a mental debate over whether or not you have the time and energy to exercise, get up and start moving!

CHAPTER THREE

Getting Ready: The Warm-Up

You've probably been hearing for years how important it is to warm up properly before starting to exercise. No experienced dancer or athlete would think of jumping into a vigorous workout without first preparing her body for the effort. Yet beginners are often so anxious to get started on their routines that they're tempted to skip the preliminaries, and even some more advanced exercise buffs still aren't clear on how to warm up properly. Once you understand what a warm-up is and what it does for you, I'm convinced you won't be tempted to short-change yourself.

The main purpose of a warm-up is, literally, to warm up your body: to raise your internal temperature, to dilate your blood vessels, to make your heart and lungs pump faster, and to allow plenty of oxygen-laden blood to reach your muscles. In terms of the way you feel, this increased oxygen supply translates to pure energy. It can make the difference between petering out in exhaustion ten minutes into your workout, or getting through it with power to spare.

As your muscles get warm, they become more flexible and more resistant to injury; at the same time, fluids are released in and around your joints to cushion them against shock. Instead of being jolted into action, your heart and lungs have time to gear up gradually. In fact, the warm-up acts as a signal to all your body's systems to get ready for the effort ahead. As a result, instead of reacting to exercise as you would to a negative stress, or a state of emergency, your body has time to build momentum smoothly and naturally, and to function like the high-powered machine it is.

For me, the warm-up also serves a psychological purpose, acting as an emotional buffer between my exercise time and everything else that's going on in my life. As my muscles warm up and my blood starts pumping, my mind begins to let go of outside projects, plans, and stresses, and I can start to focus intently on what my body is doing. Trying to plunge directly from a hectic day into a strenuous workout strikes me as making an unreasonable demand on my body.

One of the best ways to warm up is simply to do an easy version of whatever exercise you'll be doing during the workout itself. A runner might warm up by walking for a few minutes, then jogging slowly for a while before starting to run at her normal pace. A tennis player could go through some gentle swings with her racquet, jog in place for a few minutes, twist and stretch a bit, then volley easily before starting to play in earnest.

One popular misconception is that thorough stretching constitutes a warm-up. It doesn't, not by a long shot, but it always helps to add some gentle stretches to your other warm-up movements. The key word here is *gentle*: even during your warm-up, you should avoid ballistic—or bouncing—stretches. Stretching gently before your workout allows your muscles to work through the entire range of movements they will perform during your exercise routine. Remember that exercising tight muscles greatly increases your risk of injury. The stretches you do during your warm-up are meant only to bring your muscles to their best *existing* level of flexibility; this isn't the time to try to touch your chest to your knees if you've never gotten it past your waist before.

The six-part warm-up I demonstrate here can be used as preparation for any exercise routine, not just for your Winning Workout. If you memorize the moves, you can take them with you anywhere. But if you can't remember the routine, don't panic; just go back to the principle of doing an easier version of the sport or workout that will follow.

The Warm-Up Sequence 1.

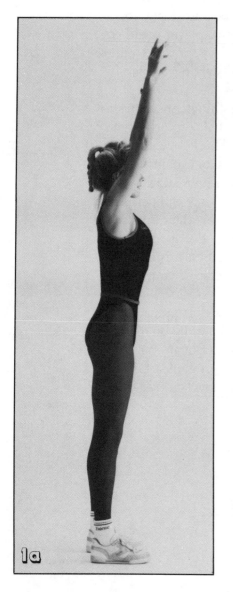

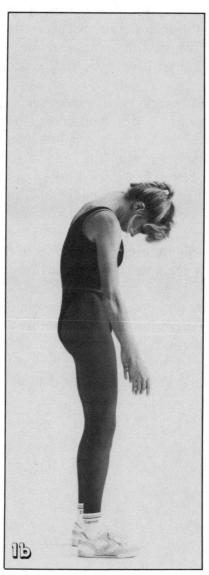

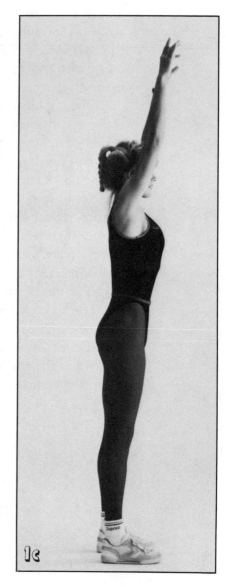

STEP 1A

Stand with your feet shoulder-width apart. Synchronize your inhalations with the lifting of your arms to the ceiling. Allow yourself six seconds to inhale deeply as you lift your arms.

STEP 1B

As you exhale, bend your knees slightly and round your *neck*.

STEP 1C

Inhale again as you reach for the ceiling.

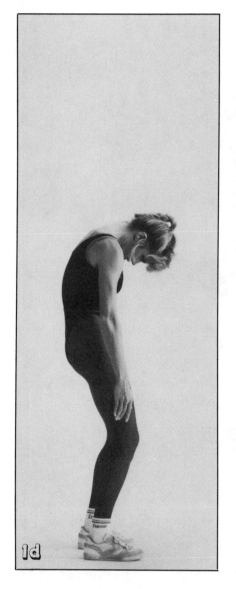

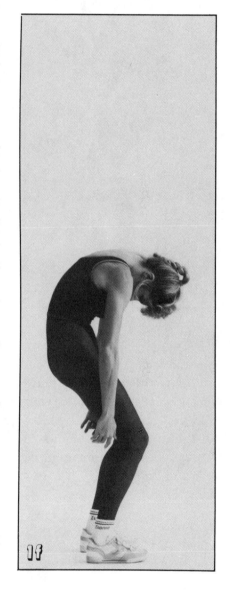

STEP 1D

As you exhale, bend your knees, drop your head, and round your *upper* back.

STEP 1E

Inhale again as you reach for the ceiling.

STEP 1F

As you exhale, bend your knees, drop your head, and round your upper and *lower* back.

★Repeat this sequence four times★

Sequence 2.

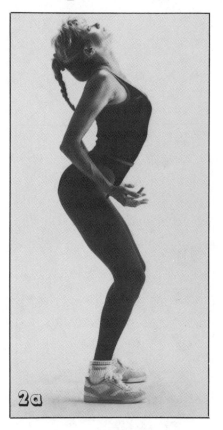

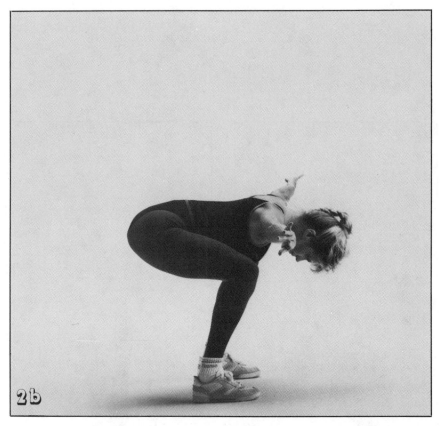

STEP 2A

Stand erect with your feet shoulder-width apart. Bend your knees as you drop your head back, push your chest forward, and pull your elbows to the rear. This action should be slow and controlled.

STEP 2B

Bend forward and ease into a parallel squat with your arms extended horizontally to the side.

Pulse or pump four times in this position.

STEP 2C

Collapse to the floor with your back rounded and your head dropped forward.

Hold four seconds.

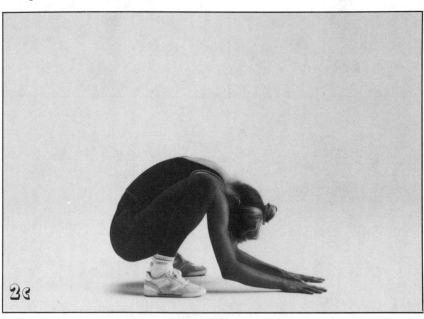

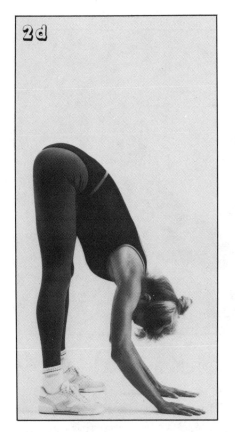

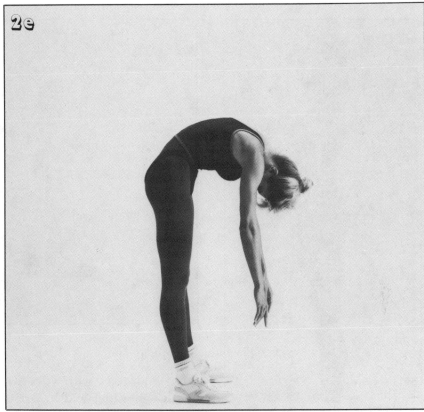

STEP 2D

Straighten your legs, maintaining contact with the floor with your hands. Depending on your flexibility, your knees may remain slightly bent. Even if you're extremely flexible, keep your knees relaxed, not locked.

STEP 2E

Straighten your back, one vertebra at a time.

★Repeat this sequence four times★

Sequence 3.

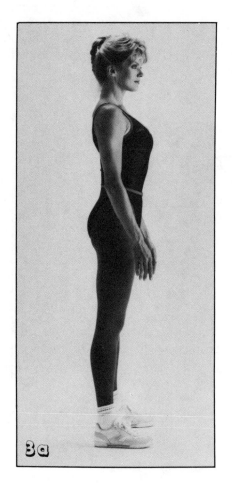

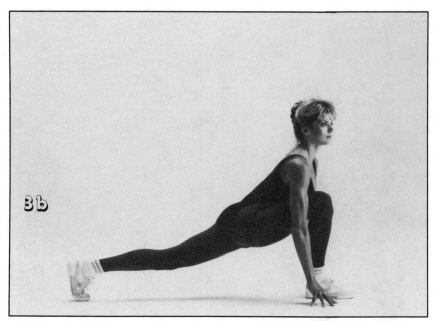

STEP 3A

Stand erect with your feet about shoulder-width apart, arms hanging naturally at your sides.

STEP 3B

With your right leg, step forward as far as you can and place your fingertips on the floor.

To protect your knees, always make sure that your bent knee is directly above or behind your toe. If your knee is extending beyond your toe, widen the distance between your legs.

Hold eight seconds.

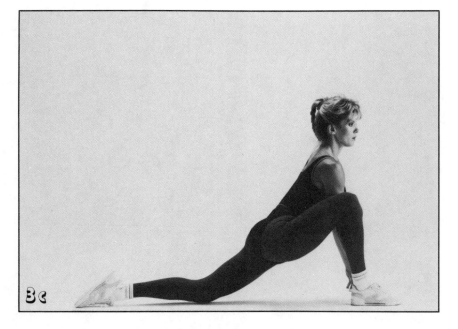

STEP 3C

Position your right shoulder inside your right thigh and touch the floor with your fingertips.

Hold 10 to 15 seconds.

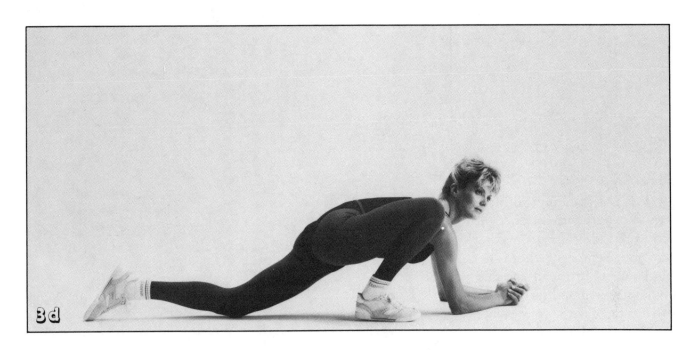

STEP 3D

Drop down until your forearms are flat on the floor.

Hold 10 to 15 seconds.

STEP 3E

Keeping your forearms flat on the floor, lift the heel of your right foot as high as you can.

Hold 10 to 15 seconds.

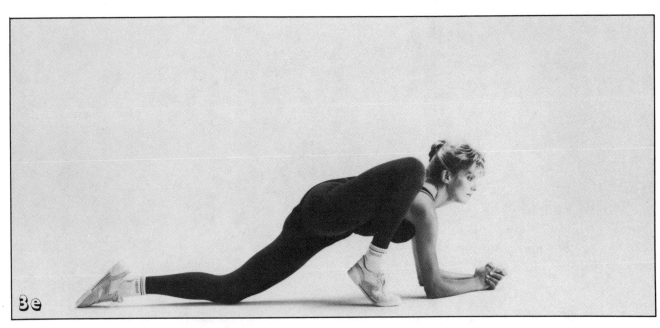

★Repeat this sequence eight times★

Then repeat the same sequence with your left leg forward

Sequence 4.

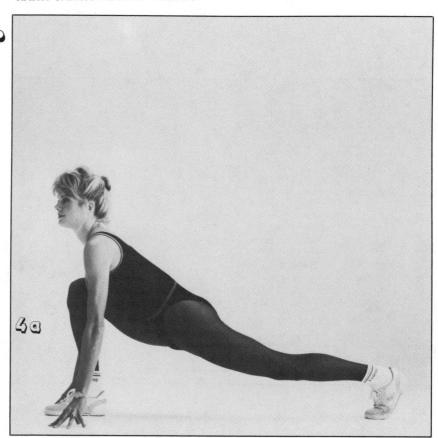

STEP 4A

From a standing position, step forward with your right foot into a deep lunge, making sure your bent right knee is behind your right toe. If you find your knee is flexed far in front of your toe, take a wider stance with your leg. Press your left hip down and forward.

Hold 10 seconds.

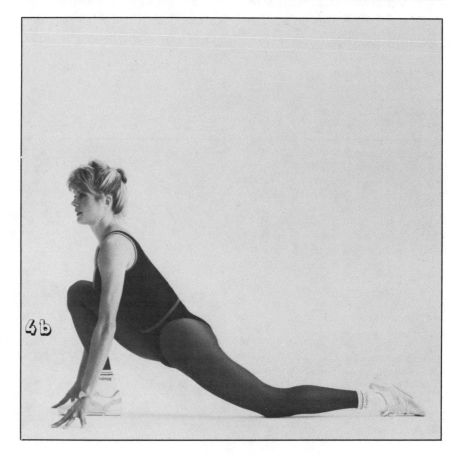

STEP 4B

With your fingertips on the floor for stability, drop your left knee to the floor and continue pressing your left hip down and forward.

Hold 10 seconds.

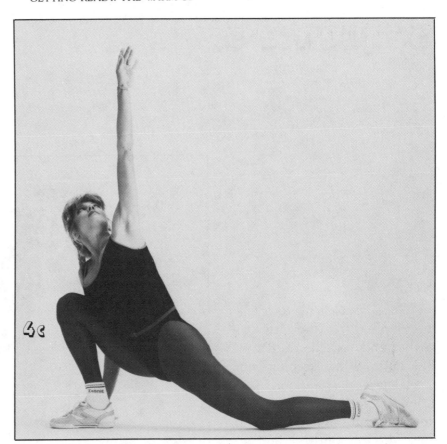

STEP 4C

Reach your left arm toward the ceiling as you rotate your head to look at your left hand.

Hold 10 seconds.

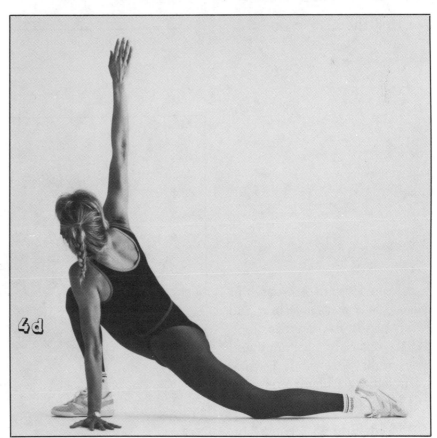

STEP 4D

Reach your right arm toward the ceiling as you rotate your head to look at your right hand.

Hold 10 seconds.

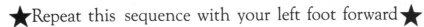

★Repeat this sequence with your left foot forward★

Sequence 5.

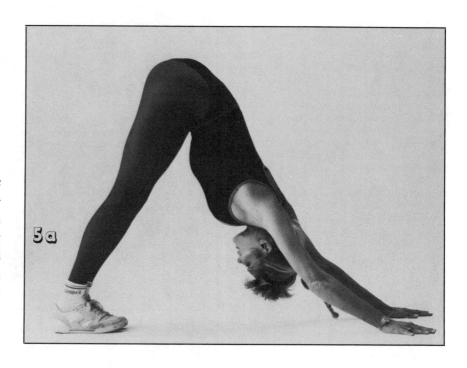

STEP 5A

Press yourself up to a pike position, with your feet together and your hands flat on the floor. While keeping your heels flat on the floor, press your shoulders down and back toward your legs. Press your lower back toward the floor.

Hold 10 to 15 seconds.

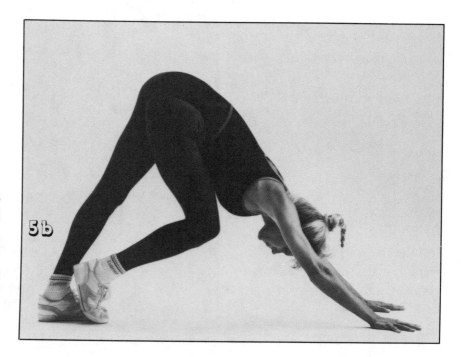

STEP 5B

Lean forward at your hips with your feet together and your hands flat on the floor. Raise your right heel and bend your right knee while keeping your left leg straight and your left heel on the floor.

Hold 10 to 15 seconds.

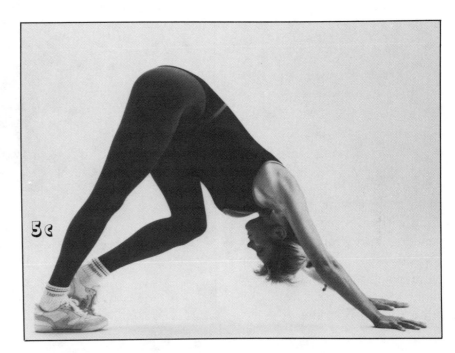

STEP 5C

Lower your right heel, straighten your right leg, raise your left heel and bend your left leg.

Hold 10 to 15 seconds.

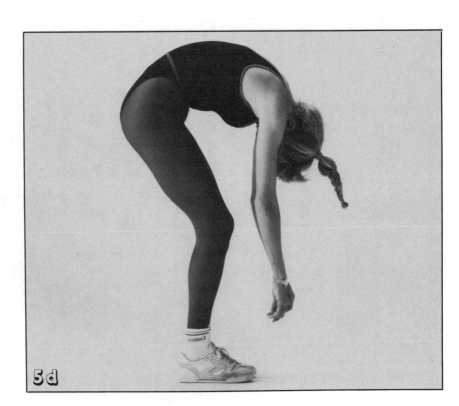

STEP 5D

Walk your hands back to your feet and roll up, one vertebra at a time.

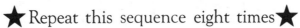

★Repeat this sequence eight times★

Sequence 6.

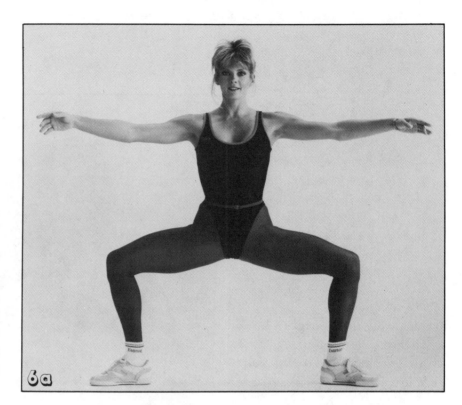

STEP 6A

Plié in a wide second position with your feet turned out, making sure your knees are directly over your toes. If you find your knees angling inside your toes, turn your feet closer to a parallel position.

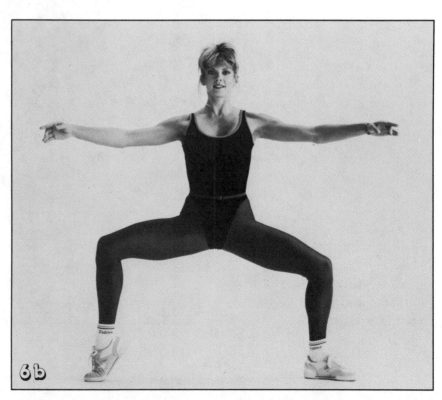

STEP 6B

Lift your right heel off the floor eight times.

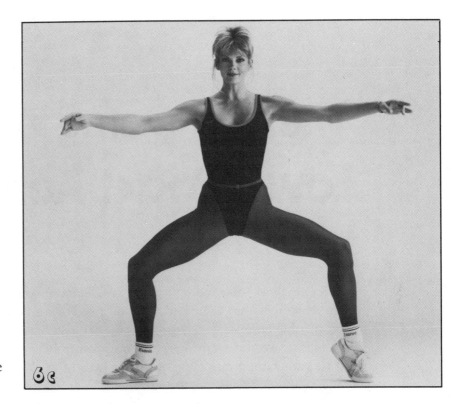

STEP 6C

Lift your left heel off the floor eight times.

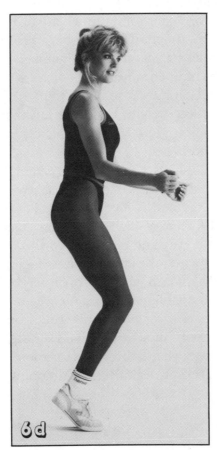

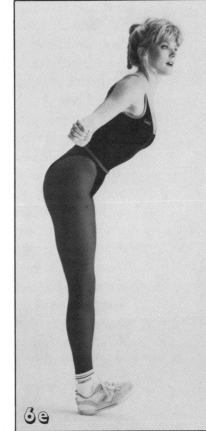

STEP 6D

Walk your feet together and rock up on your toes 16 times.

STEP 6E

Then rock back on your heels 16 times.

CHAPTER FOUR

The New Game in Town: Low-Impact Aerobics

As much as you're going to love the results of your free-weight workouts, remember that to be truly fit, you need to round out your program with aerobic exercise.

If losing weight is a priority for you, the aerobic portion of your workout is doubly important. With your free-weight workouts, you'll be building lean muscle tissue, which burns calories at a faster rate than fat tissue does, and with your aerobic routines, you'll be burning calories by expending energy. This winning combination will accelerate your weight loss dramatically, and will provide a powerful boost to your metabolism, insuring still more caloric burn-off even when you're at rest.

There are lots of good options for aerobic exercise: fast walking, jogging, running, cycling, step-climbing, swimming, jumping rope, and rowing are some of the most effective. Still, as far as I'm concerned, there's no better or more exhilarating way to boost your energy level, strengthen your heart and lungs, lose weight, and have fun than aerobic dancing. Aerobic dance makes you glow with health and vitality, and, just as important, it's never boring.

The basic idea of low-impact aerobics is to eliminate the more violent, ballistic, up-and-down movements of traditional aerobic dance—the leaps and jumps that can overstress your muscles, joints, and ligaments—without sacrificing the kind of high-energy movement that keeps your heart working within its training range. To do this, low-impact aerobics depend on the more down-to-the-ground, hip-swinging movements of jazz dance, on a gentler approach to traditional aerobic-dance steps, and (provided you're in reasonably good shape to begin with) on the use of very light wrist weights to direct more of the work load to the upper body, where there's no danger of contact with a hard surface. (If you're considerably overweight or out of shape, low-impact aerobics done *without* wrist weights provide an excellent beginner's conditioning routine.) Don't let the reference to jazz dance scare you, by the way—low-impact dance isn't a bit more complicated than traditional aerobics; it's just gentler.

Low-impact aerobic routines tend to last a bit longer than standard aerobics because they're lower-intensity workouts. But, as in all aerobic workouts, what counts is *duration*. By working a little longer within your training range, you'll get all of the same benefits. You'll burn just as many (if not more) calories, boost your circulation and your body's ability to utilize oxygen, strengthen your heart and lungs, and work up the same healthy glow and high spirits. The only things you'll miss out on are shin-splints and sore knees. I think that's a pretty good bargain, and so, apparently, do the growing numbers of low-impact aerobics fans around the country.

You'll want to check your pulse a few times during your aerobic workout to make sure you're working at your training rate. To determine your training rate, subtract your age from 220, which is the maximum number of heartbeats per minute for a healthy 10-year-old child (after the age of 10, your heartbeat begins to slow down). Multiply the results by .80, then by .60, to determine the upper and lower limits of your training rate. Your training rate can range anywhere between those two numbers. For example, if you are 30 years old, you should subtract 30 from 220 (190). Then multiply 190 by .80 ($190 \times .80 = 152$), and by .60 ($190 \times .60 = 114$). Your training rate is anywhere between 114 and 152 heartbeats per minute.

To check your heart rate, place the first two fingers of your hand (but not your thumb, which is a pulse point itself) over either the large vein on the inside of your wrist, or the carotid artery on the side of your neck, just below the jawbone. Have your watch handy, and count your heartbeats for ten seconds. Multiply the number of beats by six to find your heart rate per minute; then compare that number with your training rate.

You need to work within your training range for at least 20 to 30 minutes in order to achieve aerobic benefits. Pace yourself, though. If you're in very poor physical condition, or have never exercised before, start with only ten minutes, or whatever feels comfortable, and work your way up.

The two routines shown here should give you a pretty clear idea of what low-impact aerobic moves look like. You can use these routines as a starting point for creating your own, if you like. Or you can begin with a traditional aerobic-dance routine and make your own low-impact version simply by keeping your feet on the ground and avoiding jumps, leaps, and violent bounces.

The same kind of music you would use for standard aerobics will work fine for the low-impact variety—that is, any music that has a strong, moderately fast beat and that makes you feel good.

Make sure your workout space is well-ventilated and cleared of objects. Wear comfortable leotards and tights, or shorts and a T-shirt, and

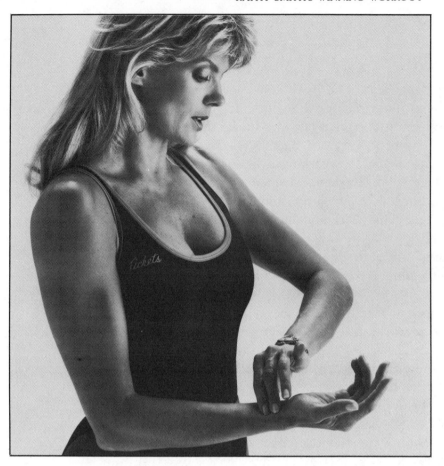

Checking Your Heart Rate At Your Wrist

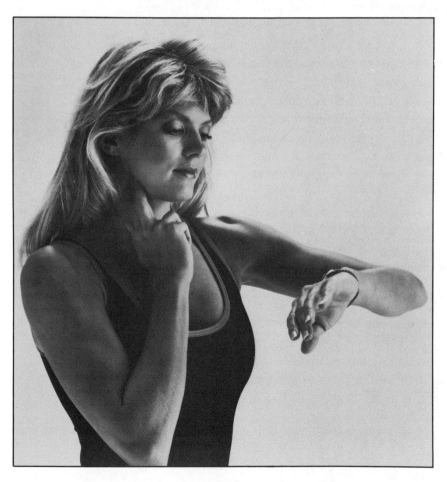

Checking Your Heart Rate At Your Neck

try to buy workout clothes that contain a large percentage of cotton so that your skin can breathe. Avoid working out on concrete or other very hard surfaces, and look for aerobic shoes that provide both cushioning and support. Although you won't be subjecting your feet to a great deal of stress, you'll still want to give them all the help they can get. And don't forget to warm up before you begin the hard stuff!

Both of the low-impact aerobics routines shown here use a traveling step as the Basic Step. In the First Routine, the Basic Step—Step Touch is used to travel forward and backward, and in the Second Routine, the Basic Step—Rocking Horse is used to travel from right to left. Each new movement is added after you've performed all the previous movements.

Begin each routine by first doing the Basic Step in place four times, then performing Movement 1 four times. Then use the Basic Step to travel backward eight steps, and repeat Movement 1 four times. Next, use the Basic Step to travel forward eight steps, repeat Movement 1 four times, and *add on* Movement 2. After you complete each backward-forward sequence, you'll be performing all your previous movements, then adding on the next movement.

Do your aerobic workout three times a week, preferably as preparation for your free-weight routine. I hope you'll give low-impact aerobics a try; but any activity, including walking, is good as long as it gets you up to your training heart rate and keeps you there for a sustained period of time. Remember, no matter what your fitness goals, your aerobic workout is essential to your training program, but if you're trying to lose weight, it's your secret weapon. If you can maintain your training rate comfortably for longer than the required 20 to 30 minutes, by all means, do so, and if you can slip in an extra half-hour of aerobics once or twice a week without feeling unduly fatigued, *go for it!*

Low-Impact Aerobics

First Routine

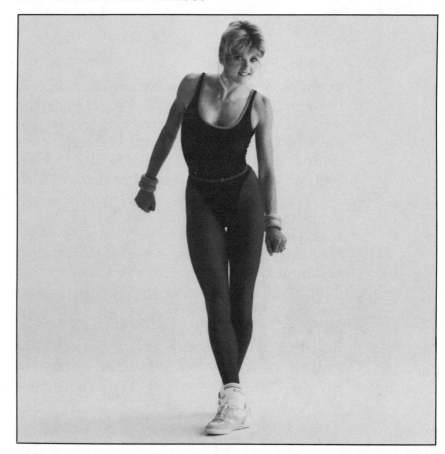

BASIC STEP. Step-Touch
A
    Step forward with your right leg directly in front of your left foot, or crossing over slightly.

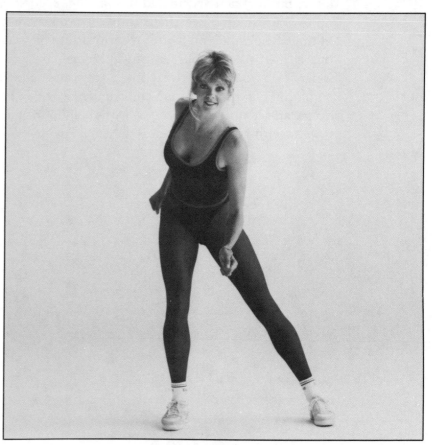

BASIC STEP B
    Transfer your weight right, and as you drop your right hip (bend your right knee and accent *down*), touch your left foot directly out to the side.

    Now step with your left foot in front of your right, transfer your weight left, and drop your left hip as you touch your right foot out to the side.

 Repeat this movement four times ★

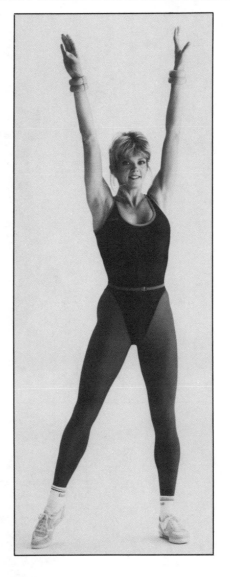
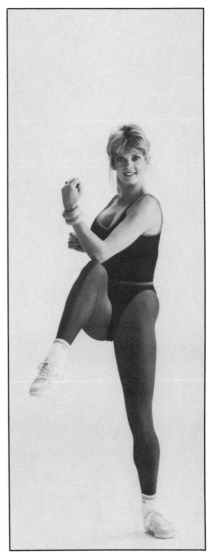

MOVEMENT 1. Elbow to Knee.

Reach your hands to the ceiling. Keeping your left foot on the ground—no bouncing—lift your right knee up as you bring your left elbow across at a diagonal to touch your knee. Return to the starting position.

Repeat, touching your left knee to your right elbow.

★ Repeat this movement four times ★

Now, using the Basic Step, step-touch backward eight steps and add the Elbow-to-Knee movement (Movement 1).

★ Repeat this sequence, but step-touch forward ★

Now add Movement 2.

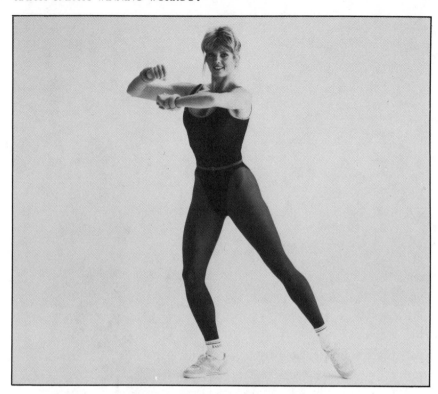

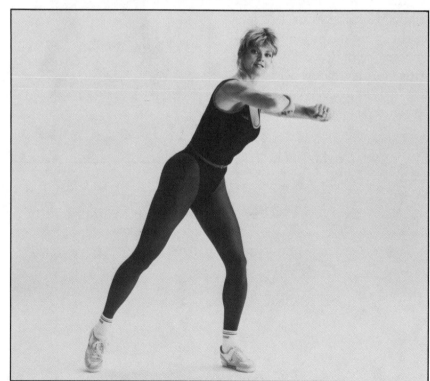

MOVEMENT 2. Lunge with Rotating Arms.

Holding your arms at chest level, lunge to the right and circle your arms around one another.

Repeat, lunging to the left.

★Repeat this movement four times★

Now, using the Basic Step, step-touch backward eight steps; add the Elbow-to-Knee movement; and add the Lunge with Rotating Arms (Movement 2).

★Repeat this sequence, but step-touch forward★

Now add Movement 3.

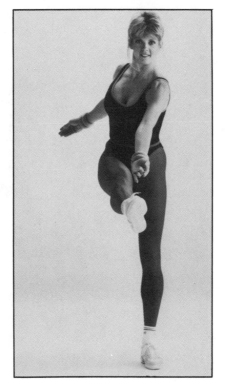 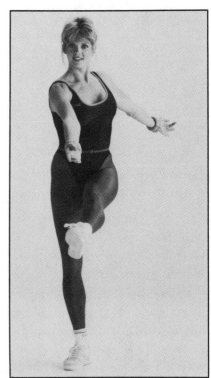

MOVEMENT 3. Low Kick.

Kick your right leg forward at a 45° angle as you reach forward with your left arm toward your right foot. Keep your left leg planted on the ground—no bouncing.

Repeat, kicking your left leg forward.

★Repeat this movement four times★

Now, using the Basic Step, step-touch backward eight steps; add the Elbow-to-Knee movement; add the Lunge with Rotating Arms; and add Low Kick (Movement 3).

★Repeat this sequence, but step-touch forward★

59

Now add Movement 4.

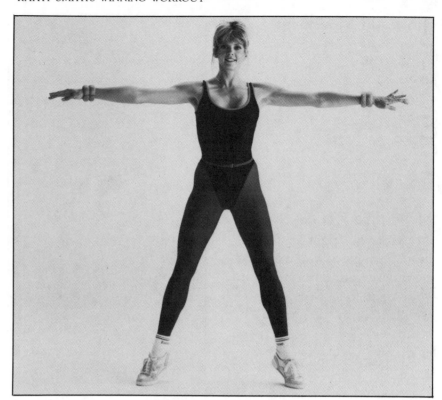

MOVEMENT 4. In-Out

4A

Step out to the side, first with your right foot, then with your left, in quick succession. (Don't move both feet out at the same time, as for a Jumping Jack.) Extend your right arm out to the side as you step out on your right foot, and extend your left arm as you step out on your left foot.

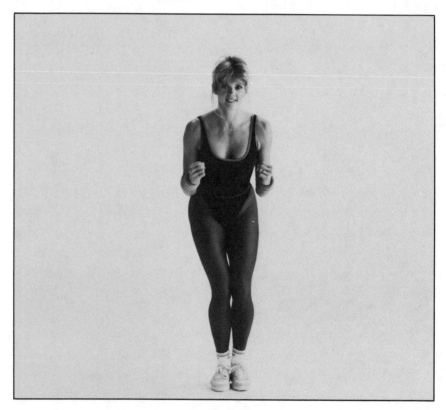

4B

Now step together, first with your right leg, then your left, again in quick succession as you drop down, bending your knees and hips slightly, and pulling your elbows and hands close to your body.

★Repeat this movement four times★

Now, using the Basic Step, step-touch backward eight steps; add the Elbow-to-Knee movement; add the Lunge with Rotating Arms; add the Low Kick; and add the In-Out (Movement 4).

★Repeat this sequence, but step-touch forward★

Low-Impact Aerobics Second Routine

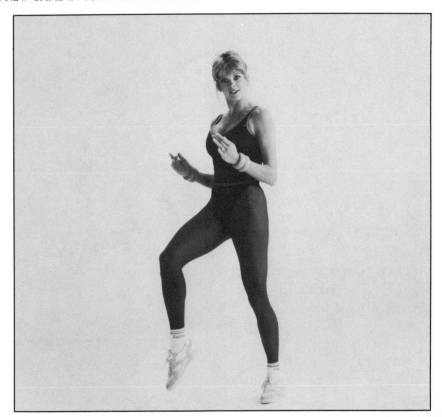

BASIC STEP. Rocking Horse

A

Moving to the right, transfer your weight to your left foot as you lean backward, bending your elbows and keeping your hands close to your chest.

BASIC STEP B

Now rock forward onto your right foot as you unfold your arms and extend them back, and as you lift your left leg off the floor.

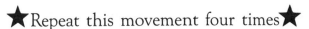 ★Repeat this movement four times★

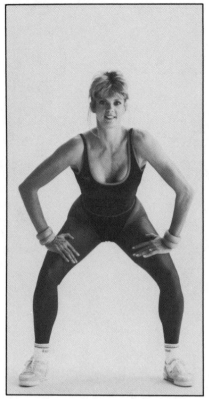

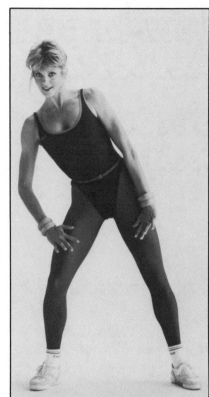

MOVEMENT 1. Down-Up.

1A

Place your hands on your thighs as you squat, bending forward at your hips.

1B

Press up and to the right, keeping your knees slightly bent.

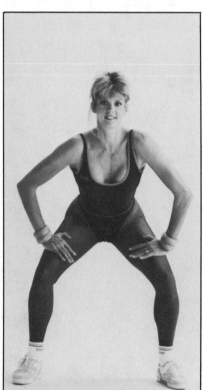

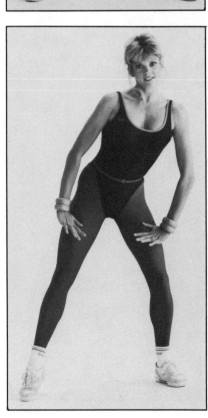

1C

Drop back down to a squat.

1D

Press up and to the left, keeping your knees slightly bent.

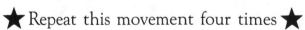

★ Repeat this movement four times ★

Now repeat the basic Rocking Horse step, stepping to the right eight steps, and add Down-Up movement (Movement 1A through 1D).

★ Repeat this sequence, stepping to the left. ★

Now add Movement 2.

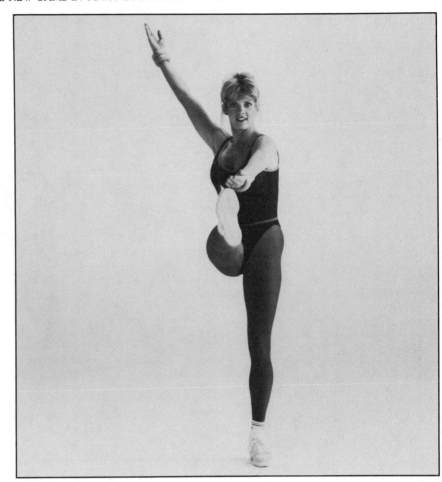

MOVEMENT 2. High Kick.

Kick your right leg forward at a 45° to 90° angle as you reach forward with your left arm toward your right foot.

Repeat, kicking your left leg forward.

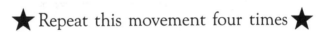 ★Repeat this movement four times★

Now repeat the basic Rocking Horse step, stepping to the right eight steps; add Down-Up movement; and add High Kick movement (Movement 2).

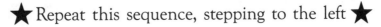 ★Repeat this sequence, stepping to the left★

Now add Movement 3.

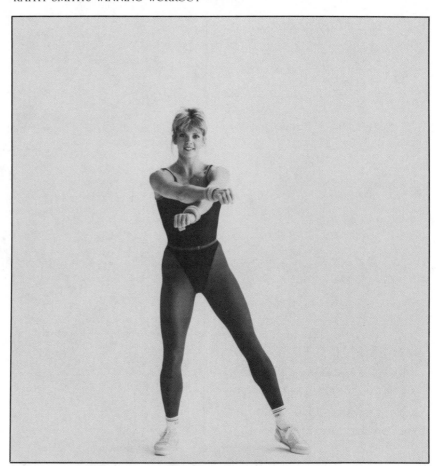

MOVEMENT 3. Arm Cross
with Rocking Hips.
3A Holding your arms straight,
cross them in front of you and
rock your hips right and left.

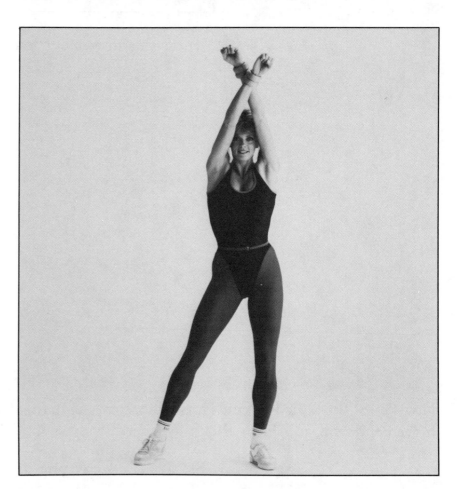

3B
Start with your arms low,
and progressively raise them for
four counts.

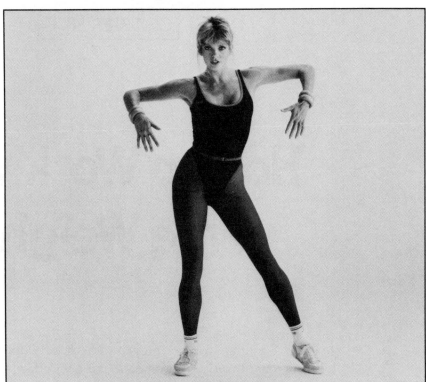

3C

Continue to rock your hips, but open your arms, drop them, and shake out your hands.

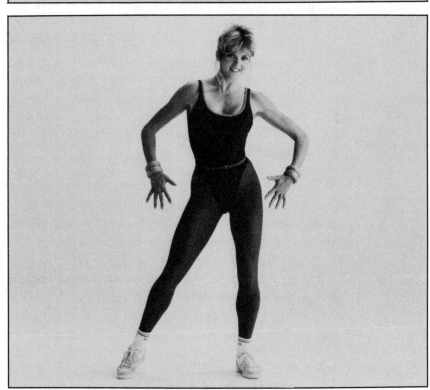

3D

Continue to rock your hips as you concentrate on letting your hands hang loose, shaking them out.

★Repeat this movement four times★

Now repeat the basic Rocking Horse step, stepping to the right eight steps; add Down-Up movement; add High Kick movement; and add Arm Cross with Rocking Hips (Movement 3).

★Repeat this sequence, stepping to the left★

CHAPTER FIVE

How to Work with Free Weights

The Winning Workout program wasn't developed for hardcore body builders, but for ordinary women looking for a fast, effective shape-up, so I'm not going to ask you to absorb a lot of esoteric anatomical information or strange jargon.

All you'll need to know for now are a few key terms and some basic principles that will give you an understanding of what you'll be doing and why. By the time you've gone through the workouts a few times, you'll be thoroughly familiar with most of them.

REPETITION: (also known as a "rep") one complete exercise; for example, one bicep curl or one sit-up.

SET: a group of repetitions; for example, eight bicep curls. During the program, you'll be performing one, two, or three *sets* each consisting of a given number of *reps*. Three *sets* of eight *reps* means eight repetitions for an exercise, performed three times.

Although you shouldn't rest between *reps*, it's important to rest for a minute or two between *sets*, so that after thoroughly tiring a muscle group, you can relax it before proceeding. This will allow your muscles to refuel with oxygen and rid themselves of lactic acid buildup, so that they can undertake the next effort without strain.

PROGRESSIVE OVERLOAD: the basic tenet of all resistance exercise. This is also the principle that allows free-weight training to produce such dramatic improvements in muscle strength and tone.

When muscles are stimulated by being overloaded—by being asked to do more work than they're accustomed to—they respond by becoming stronger. But once they've adapted to the new level of stimulation, they need to be overloaded again before they'll improve further. As a result, weight training is a process of reaching, then transcending, a series of plateaus. In terms of your workouts, this means that whenever a particular work load becomes easy for you, it's time to move on to the next level of overload.

We use the terms *progressive overload* and *progressive resistance* because overloading is done in small increments, in order to continually challenge the muscles without exhausting or injuring them.

There are several different ways to overload a muscle, some of which produce results that are of interest only to competitive body builders or weight lifters. The two most common methods are to increase the amount of weight being lifted, and to increase the number of times you lift that weight. The first method tends to increase muscle strength, while the second tends to increase muscle endurance. Since both are important to a well-conditioned body, I've incorporated both methods into your program.

Basic Equipment

Your equipment for the Winning Workout program should consist of a barbell, dumbbells, and a bench. You might also want to add ankle and/or wrist weights to use in your aerobic workouts, or to add heft to a standard exercise routine. All told, your entire investment will still be very reasonable, certainly no more than it would cost to outfit yourself for most other sports.

A barbell is a long bar with weights attached to both ends. You adjust the total weight of the barbell by changing the weights at each end. A dumbbell is a short bar with weights at both ends, and is usually used in pairs, one held in each hand. Not all dumbbells are adjustable, but I advise you to find ones that are, unless you plan to devote a lot of storage space to several sets of dumbbells of different weights. If you do buy the adjustable type, make sure the weights can be changed easily and fastened securely to the ends of the dumbbells.

Throughout this book, I'm working with my own line of IN'TONE weights. I designed these to eliminate certain problems that had irritated me when I worked with standard men's weights. For example, the IN'TONE Hideawayts—the barbell and dumbbell you see in the photos—are more comfortable to hold, with rubber bumpers to protect your fingers and the floor. Each weight cylinder fits inside the others, so they're more compact than standard weights. I must confess, I also designed them to look more feminine than traditional weights, but that's just a matter of personal taste. Don't let the unusual appearance of my weights throw you; they're the same basic weight-training equipment I've been describing, and any weights you feel comfortable working with will be fine.

Beginners are often tempted to skip the bench. My advice is: *don't*. An adequate bench costs surprisingly little, and trying to improvise with a table or chair will throw off your form in many weight-training exercises. It's helpful to have a benchpress bench (one that allows you to rest your barbell on steel supports at one end), but it isn't essential.

What to Wear

The same clothes you wear for your aerobic workouts are fine; you can add sweats or a warm-up suit if you're in a chilly environment. Any sneakers are suitable.

When to Work Out

Work out every other day, three times a week. Don't try to accelerate your shape-up by working out every day; your muscles need at least 48 hours of rest between workouts to rid themselves of toxins and to allow for the progressive overload principle to have its effect. You *can* do abdominal exercises every day, since these muscles respond well to continual exercise, but stick to the recommended schedule for the rest of the program.

As I mentioned earlier, it's a good idea to do your free-weight workout right after your aerobic workout, rather than doing them on alternate days. This will allow your body to rest and recuperate thoroughly between exercise sessions.

There is no "best" time to exercise. It depends entirely on your schedule and your personal preference. I love to work out early in the morning, but if you're the type of person who can't even speak before 11 a.m., by all means schedule your workouts in the evening. *Do* try to exercise at the same time each day. A schedule will help you maintain a routine, and make it easier for your family and friends to accommodate it. Don't schedule workouts for at least two full hours after you eat a meal, or within two hours of going to bed. The first will interfere with your digestion, and the second will leave you too stimulated to fall asleep.

Finding the Right Weight

There is no scientific way to determine how many pounds you should lift in a given exercise; it's matter of your own body structure and conditioning. Some women find five pounds much too light for arm exercises, while others can barely get through a set at this weight.

The best way to decide what works for you is by experimenting. Pick up a weight that feels comfortable and go through one set of reps. If you feel that you could easily do more repetitions at the end of the set, the weight is too light for you. If you can't make it through the set, the weight is too heavy. If you've found the right weight, your muscles will feel fatigued but not strained by the end of the set.

As you begin, I'd rather you erred in the direction of too little weight than too much. Start with a relatively light weight, and if that proves *too* light, move to a heavier weight on your next set. It won't take long for you to develop a sure sense of what's right for the various muscle groups in your body.

Using the Proper Form

Learning the proper form for your weight-training exercises isn't difficult, and it's essential if you're to get the full benefit of this or any weight-training program. To insure that you're doing the exercises correctly, I want you to go through each of them the first time *without using any weights at all.*

Observing yourself in a mirror, do each exercise just as it appears in the photos. Check frequently to be sure your position matches mine as closely as possible. Don't skip the details: if my arms are slightly bent in one of the exercises, check to see that yours aren't straight or *very* bent. If my shoulders are down and relaxed, make sure that yours are, too.

Only when you feel confident that you understand the technique should you go ahead and perform the exercise with light weights. Don't rush the learning process. Remember, weight training stresses the muscles in a very specific, concentrated way. If you put that stress where it's not needed, you're not going to get the same rewards, and you'll probably wake up with stiff muscles the next morning.

Try to make all your movements smooth and controlled, not rushed or jerky. In weight training, the lowering portion of an exercise, called the negative phase, is just as important as the lifting, or positive phase. The exercise isn't complete until you've lifted the weights smoothly through your full range of motion, paused for a moment at the top, and lowered the weight, just as smoothly and with just as much control, to your starting point.

Finally, it's very important to keep breathing throughout all the exercises. Breathing normally and rhythmically will help your movements flow more smoothly and will keep your energy level high. By contrast, holding your breath will raise your blood pressure and make you feel fatigued very quickly. The rule of thumb most weight trainers follow is to exhale on the positive, or lifting, phase of the exercise, and inhale on the negative, or lowering phase. But if you have trouble adapting to this rhythm, don't worry about it; just keep breathing in whatever way feels most natural to you.

As a safety precaution, if you feel unsure about any of the exercises in this program (especially those using a barbell), you may wish to have a training partner observe the first few times you do an exercise and help you put the weights in place before you lift them.

If this seems like a lot to remember, don't panic. Use the photos and instructions to guide you. After a couple of workouts, you'll feel like a pro.

Workout Chart

This chart will give you a record of your lifting program. A space is provided for you to enter the amount of weight you are lifting in each exercise each week. This weight should be increased as your program progresses. A space is also provided for you to note the number of repetitions you do in each set. Remember, one of your objectives is to set goals at the beginning and strive to achieve them.

Exercise	Reps	Sets	Weight/Repetitions	Wt. / Reps.
Date				

CHAPTER SIX

Winning Workout: Phase 1

Your Winning Workouts are divided into three phases. Each phase works the muscles of your entire body, but each is designed to give you maximum benefits for your level of conditioning.

You'll spend four weeks working out in each Phase, during which time you'll progessively overload your muscles by gradually increasing the number of repetitions of each exercise. For example, if the instructions for an exercise indicate eight to twelve repetitions, you'll start by doing eight at a comfortable weight, then increase to nine repetitions at your next workout, then ten, and so on.

In most cases, I've allowed a little leeway in the number of repetitions, so that if you work out three times a week, you can remain at a given number of repetitions for an extra workout or two, or do the maximum number at your last two workouts. This allows you to proceed at a comfortable pace. If you're having an off day, or finding a number of repetitions particularly challenging, stick with the number of reps you did at your last workout. Your body is telling you that you're not yet ready to move on.

By the third week of Phase 1, you'll move up to two sets of reps for each exercise. At this point, you'll go back to doing the minimum number of reps for each set: if you're asked to do eight to twelve reps, start by doing two sets of eight reps each, then move to two sets of nine reps each, then ten, and so on.

Follow the sequence and progression indicated for all of the exercises. Please don't skip around or try to jump ahead. If you're already fairly strong when you start the program, you can simply use more weight for the exercises than someone who is not as strong, but don't try to ad lib. There is a reason for everything in a good weight-training program, and this one was very carefully planned to give you maximum toning in a relatively short period of time. Don't try to rush anything. You'll need the full

12 weeks, not only to tone and reshape your muscles, but to allow your body's infrastructure—your tendons, ligaments, and internal organs—to adjust to the strengthening process taking place outside.

Give yourself three or four workout sessions just to become thoroughly comfortable with the exercises. They've been set up to give you head-to-toe conditioning at a beginner level, but they're not beginner exercises per se. You'll be doing these same exercises—or tougher versions of them—for as long as you continue working with free weights, so you might as well learn to do them correctly right from the start.

That's it for the do's and don'ts. Now let's get started. And remember, this isn't life-or-death stuff—have fun with it!

Winning Workout / Phase 1

EXERCISE	REPETITIONS	THIGHS	BUTTOCKS	HIPS	QUADS	LOWER BACK	HAM-STRINGS	CALVES
1. Step-Ups	15 for each leg	X	X	X				
2. Dumbbell squats	12 to 15		X	X	X	X		
3. Lunges on box	12 to 15 for each leg, alternating legs		X		X		X	
4. Calf raises	15 to 20							X
5. Barbell bench presses	8 to 12							
6. Barbell bent rows	8 to 12							
7. Seated press— behind the neck	8 to 12							
8. Dumbbell bicep curls	8 to 12 for each arm							
9. Dumbbell wrist curls	12 to 15 for each wrist							
10. Reverse sit-ups	20 to 30							
11. Seated twists	20 to 30 on each side							

*Week 1 and Week 2: one set
Week 3 and Week 4: two sets

PECTORALS	DELTOIDS	TRICEPS	LATS	BICEPS	SPINAL ERECTORS	TRAPEZIUS	FOREARMS	ABDOM-INALS	INTERNAL OBLIQUE	EXTERNAL OBLIQUE	WAIST
X	X	X									
			X	X	X	X					
	X	X									
				X							
							X				
								X			X
									X	X	X

Summary of Repetitions/ Phase 1

	Week 1	Week 2	Week 3	Week 4	
	1 set	1 set	2 sets	2 sets	
UPPER BODY	8 to 10	10 to 12	8 to 10	10 to 12	Repetitions
LOWER BODY	12 to 13	13 to 15	8 to 10	10 to 12	Repetitions
ABDOMINALS AND OBLIQUES	20 to 30	20 to 30	30 to 40	30 to 40	Repetitions

Exercise 1.

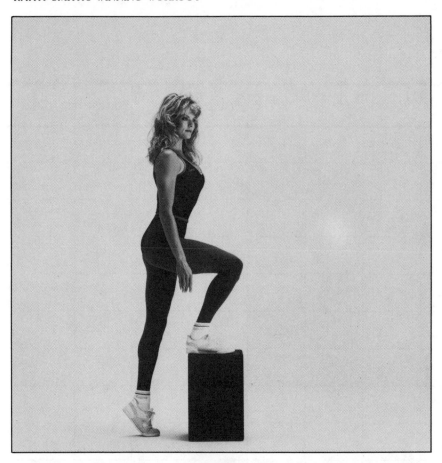

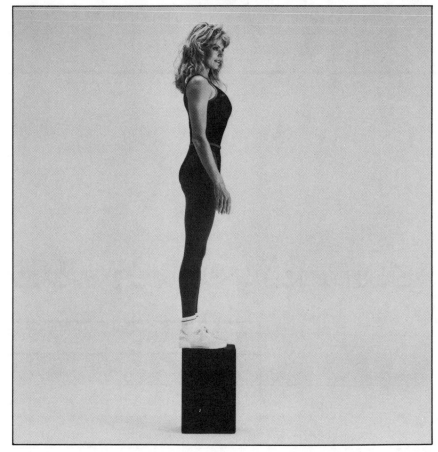

EXERCISE 1. Step-Ups.

Use a sturdy box or bench about 16″ to 18″ high.

1A

Place one foot on the box.

1B

Step up onto the box as you exhale, without pushing off with your other leg.

1C

Return to the starting position as you inhale.

★Repeat this exercise 15 times for each leg, alternating legs★

Exercise 2.

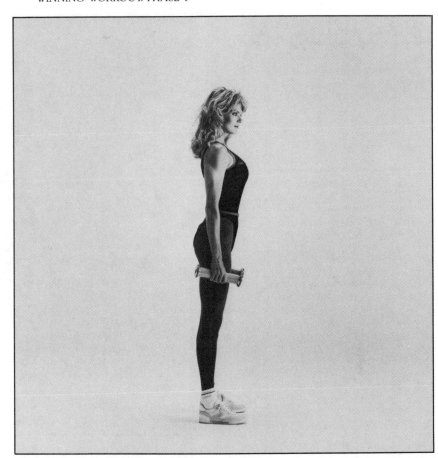

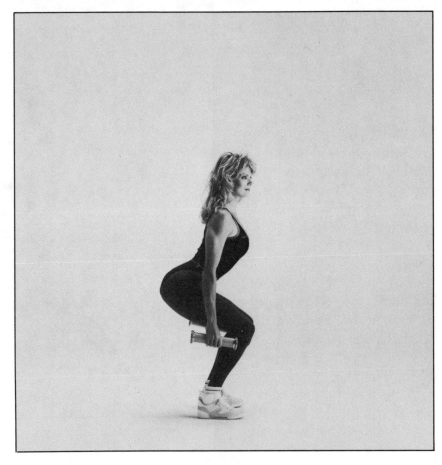

EXERCISE 2. Dumbbell Squats.

Stand with your feet apart, holding a dumbbell in each hand, with your arms hanging by your sides.

2A

Extend your arms forward. While keeping your feet flat, inhale and squat until your thighs are parallel to the floor. Keep your back straight.

2B

Exhale as you return to the starting position.

If you lack ankle flexibility, raise your heels by standing on a 2″ by 4″ board, with the balls of your feet on the floor.

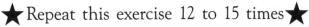 ★Repeat this exercise 12 to 15 times★

Exercise 3.

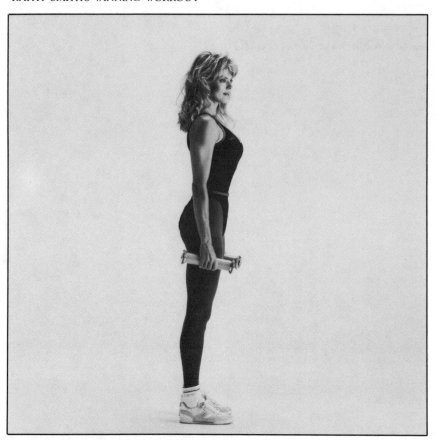

EXERCISE 3. Lunges on Box.

Stand erect, holding a dumbbell in each hand. Position a 16″ or 18″ box or bench against the wall so it won't tip or shift.

3A

Step forward, placing one foot on the box. Keep your rear leg straight and your rear foot flat. Exhale as you step.

3B

Return to the starting position as you inhale.

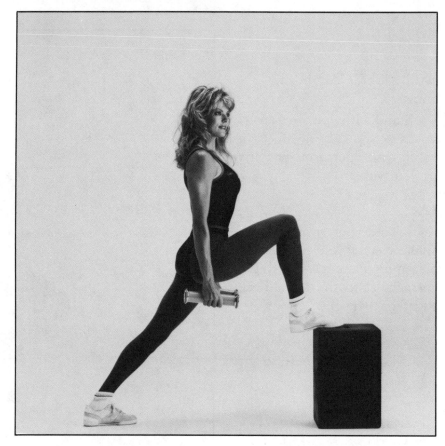

★Repeat this exercise 12 to 15 times for each leg, alternating legs★

Exercise 4.

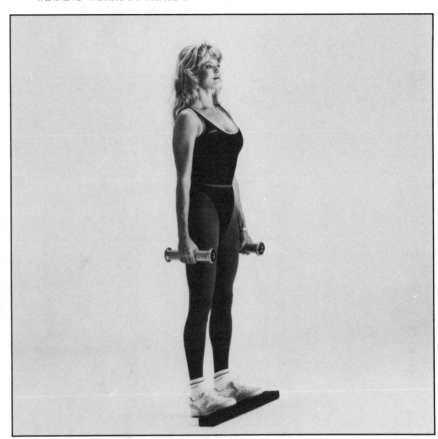

EXERCISE 4. Calf Raises.

Stand erect, holding a dumbbell in each hand. Place the balls of your feet on a 2″ block, with your heels touching the floor. Breathe normally throughout this exercise.

4A

Rise high on your tiptoes while keeping your knees straight.

4B

Lower your heels to the starting position.

You may vary this exercise by turning your toes out or in.

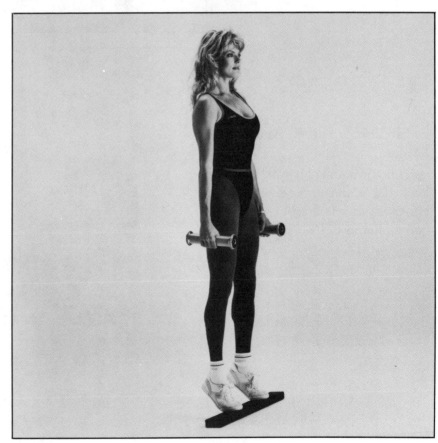

★ Repeat this exercise 15 to 20 times ★

Exercise 5.

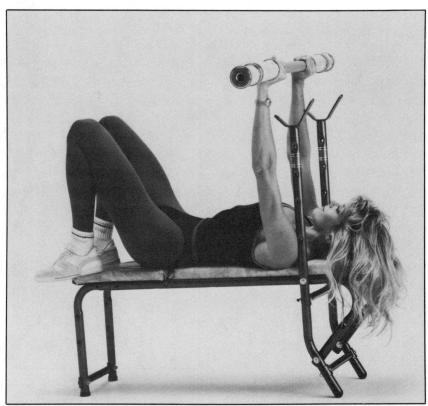

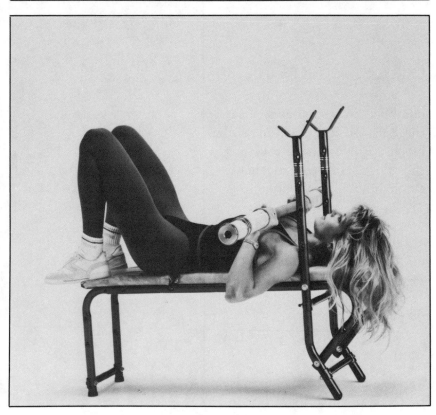

EXERCISE 5. Barbell Bench Presses.

Lie on the bench with your back flat and your feet resting either flat on the floor or on the bench. Remove the barbell from the support racks and hold it at arm's length overhead.

5A

Lower the barbell to your chest as you inhale.

5B

Straighten your arms, pressing the barbell to the ceiling as you exhale.

★Repeat this exercise eight to 12 times★

Exercise 6.

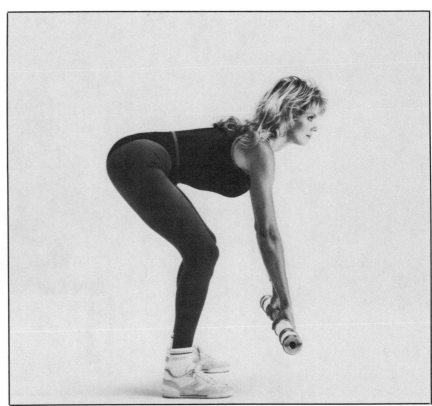

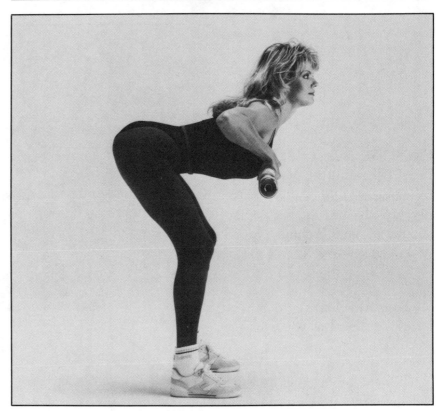

EXERCISE 6. Barbell Bent Rows.

Grasp the barbell with an "over-grip," palms facing downward, hands shoulder-width apart. Lean forward from your hips, keeping your back flat and your knees bent. Arms are extended downward.

6A

As you exhale, pull the barbell upward until it touches your chest.

6B

Lower the barbell to the starting position as you inhale.

★Repeat this exercise eight to 12 times★

Exercise 7.

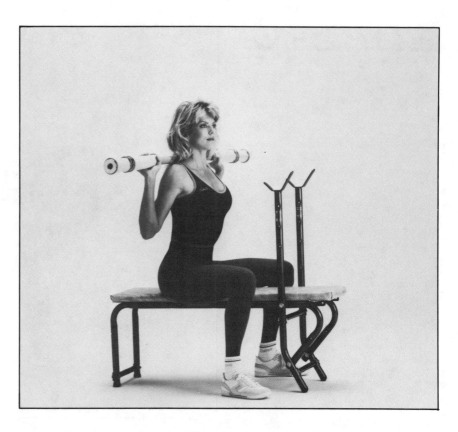

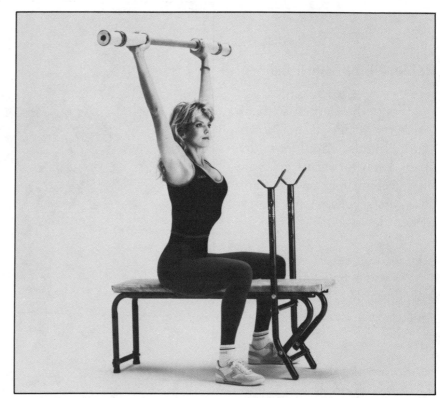

EXERCISE 7. Seated Presses—Behind the Neck.

Sit astride the bench, holding the barbell across your shoulders and behind your neck, using a wide grip.

7A

Press the barbell to arm's length overhead as you exhale.

7B

Lower the barbell to the starting position as you inhale.

★Repeat this exercise eight to 12 times★

Exercise 8.

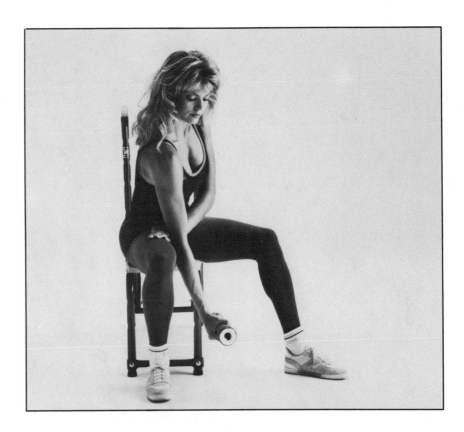

EXERCISE 8. Dumbbell Bicep Curls.

Sit on the end of the bench with your feet wide apart. Grasp one dumbbell in your right hand with an "under-grip," palm facing upward. Position your right arm straight down, with your right elbow resting against the inside of your right thigh.

8A

Exhale as you slowly curl the dumbbell as far as possible, keeping the back of your upper right arm against your left forearm.

8B

Inhale as you lower the dumbbell and return to the starting position.

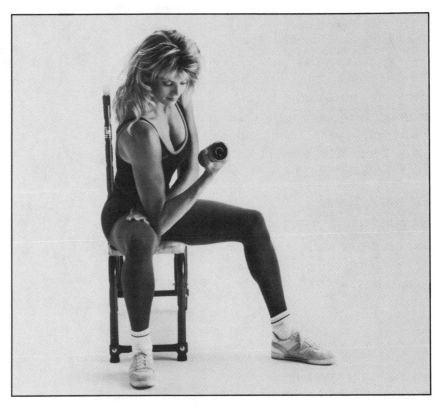

★Repeat this exercise eight to 12 times★

Exercise 9.

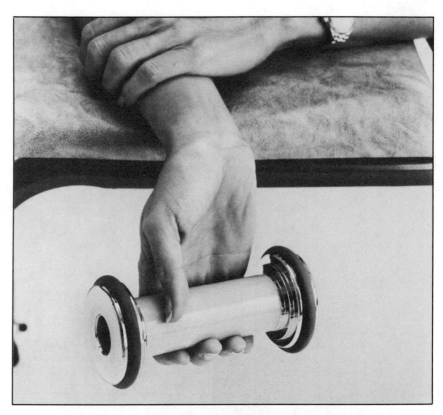

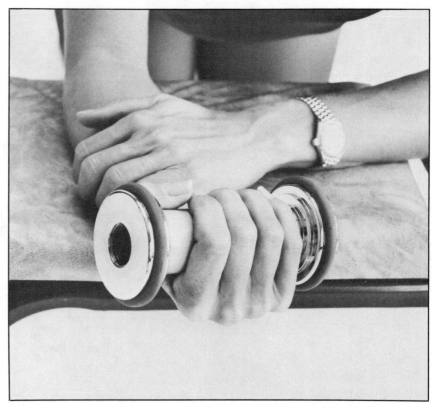

EXERCISE 9. Dumbbell Wrist Curls.

Rest your right forearm along the top of the bench, grasping the dumbbell with an "under-grip," palm facing upward. Bend your wrist downward as far as you can.

9A

Grip the dumbbell firmly and bend your wrist upward as far as you can without allowing your forearms to leave the bench.

9B

Lower the dumbbell as far as you can, returning to the starting position.

★ Repeat this exercise eight to 12 times ★

Exercise 10.

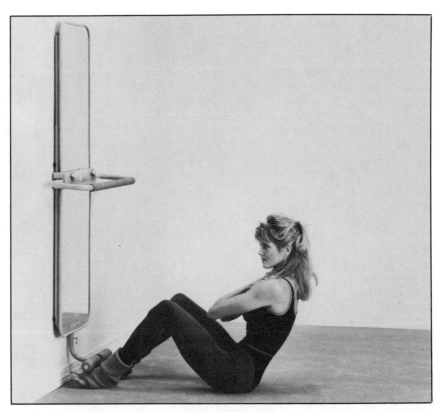

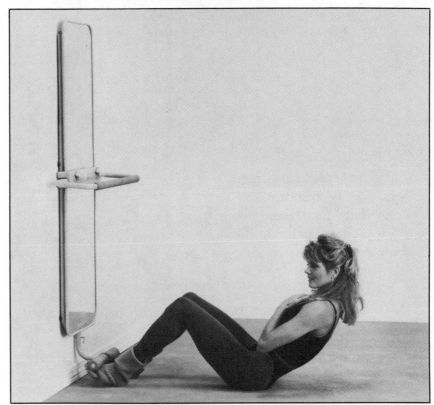

EXERCISE 10. Reverse Sit-Ups.

Sit with your knees bent and your arms crossed over your chest. Secure your feet if necessary.

10A

Lie halfway back as you exhale.

10B

Raise yourself to the starting position as you inhale.

★Repeat this exercise 20 to 30 times★

85

Exercise 11.

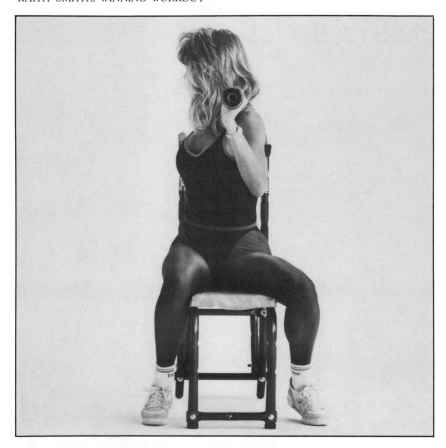

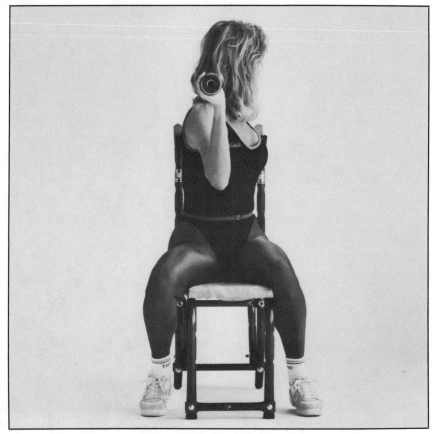

EXERCISE 11. Seated Twists.

Sit at the end of the bench, and place the barbell comfortably on your shoulders with your feet planted firmly on the floor for stability.

11A

Keep your hips facing forward as you rotate first to the right . . .

11B

. . . then to the left.

★Repeat this exercise 20 to 30 times★

Now do the Cool-Down and Stretch described in Chapter 9.

CHAPTER SEVEN

Winning Workout: Phase 2

Congratulations! In just four weeks, you've made it to the second level of your program! By now you should feel like an old hand at weight training, so for the next four weeks, I want you to work on perfecting your form and increasing your concentration at each workout. It's time to start polishing your act!

You'll notice that I've added some new exercises to this phase of the program, and toughened some of the ones you've been doing for the last month. They're all well within your capability at this point, and you'll enjoy the challenge. Remember to first run through each new exercise a few times without weights to be sure you're directing the effort exactly where you want it before you ask your muscles to kick in.

In Phase 2, you'll begin by doing two sets of reps for each exercise for the first two weeks, then move on to three sets for the last two weeks. Unless you find yourself breezing through the second week of Phase 2 with very little effort, stick with the weights you used in Phase 1. If you feel you must add poundage at that point, do so in very small increments.

Midway through Phase 2, you should feel markedly better than you did when you began the program, and you'll also begin to see changes in your overall appearance.

It's very important to use your motivation and relaxation techniques throughout this period, since the midway point of any undertaking can make us feel impatient to reach the finish line. Focus on what you've already achieved, and how much better you already feel. Emphasize the positive, and I promise you: you'll get your rewards!

Winning Workout / Phase 2

EXERCISE	REPETITIONS	THIGHS	BUTTOCKS	HIPS	QUADS	LOWER BACK	HAM-STRINGS	CALVES
1. Step-Ups with alternate arms	15 for each leg	X	X	X				
2. Barbell squats	12 to 15		X	X	X	X		
3. Dumbbell knee lunges	12 to 15		X		X		X	
4. Deadlifts	12 to 15						X	
5. Good-mornings	12 to 15						X	
6. One-legged calf raises	15 to 20 for each leg							X
7. Barbell bench presses	8 to 12							
8. Dumbell flies	8 to 12							
9. One-arm dumbbell bent rows	8 to 12 for each arm							
10. Upright rows	8 to 12							
11. Side lateral raises	8 to 12							
12. Barbell curls	8 to 12							
13. Tricep extensions	8 to 12 for each arm							
14. Barbell wrist curls, 2 positions	15 to 20							
15. 4-Part sit-up routine	10 cycles							
16. Reverse curl-ups	10 cycles							
17. Floor side bends	20 to 30 on each side							
18. Beginning reverse trunk twists	20 to 30 on each side							

*Week 1 and Week 2: two sets
 Week 3 and Week 4: three sets

PECTORALS	DELTOIDS	TRICEPS	LATS	BICEPS	SPINAL ERECTORS	TRAPEZIUS	FOREARMS	ABDOM-INALS	INTERNAL OBLIQUE	EXTERNAL OBLIQUE	WAIST
					X						
					X						
X	X	X									
X	X										
			X								
	X			X		X					
	X					X					
				X							
		X									
							X				
								X			X
								X			X
									X	X	X
									X	X	X

Summary of Repetitions / Phase 2

	Week 5	Week 6	Week 7	Week 8	
	2 sets	2 sets	3 sets	3 sets	
UPPER BODY	8 to 10	10 to 12	8 to 10	10 to 12	Repetitions
LOWER BODY	12 to 13	13 to 15	12 to 13	13 to 15	Repetitions
ABDOMINALS AND OBLIQUES	20 to 30	20 to 30	30 to 40	30 to 40	Repetitions

Exercise 1.

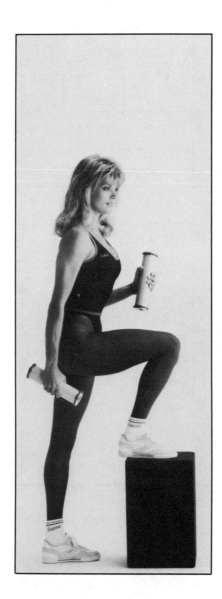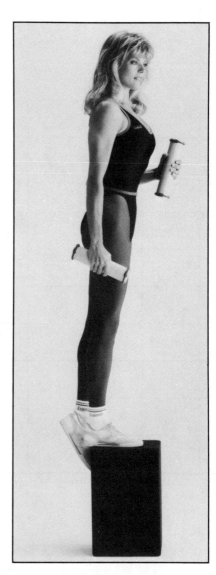

EXERCISE 1. Step-Ups with Alternate Arms.

Hold a dumbbell in each hand and use a sturdy box or bench about 16″ to 18″ high.

1A

Place your right foot flat on the box, and raise the left dumbbell until your left arm is parallel to the floor.

1B

Step up onto the box as you exhale, without pushing off with your left leg. Return to the starting position as you inhale and lower your left arm.

1C

Place your left foot on the box, and raise the right dumbbell until your right arm is parallel to the floor.

1D

Step up onto the box as you exhale without pushing off with your right leg. Return to the starting position as you inhale and lower your right arm.

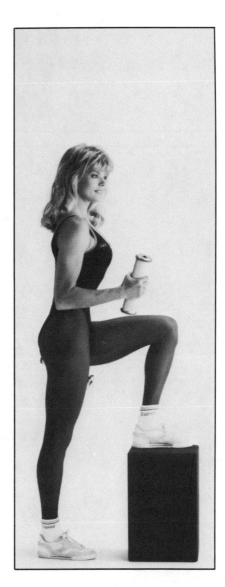 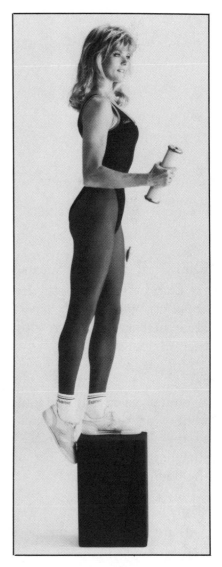

★Repeat this exercise 15 times for each leg, alternating legs★

Exercise 2.

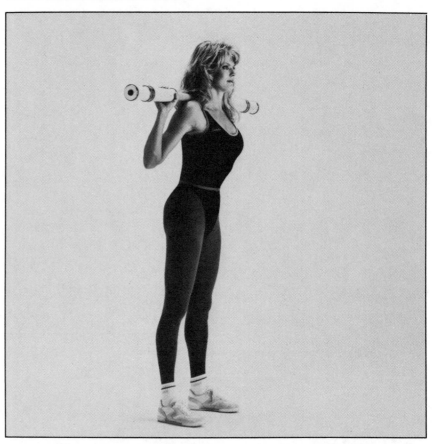

EXERCISE 2. Barbell Squats.

Stand erect with your feet about shoulder-width apart. Place the barbell low across the back of your shoulders.

2A

Inhale vigorously and squat until your thighs are parallel to the floor. Keep your back straight and your feet flat on the floor.

2B

Return to the starting position as you exhale.

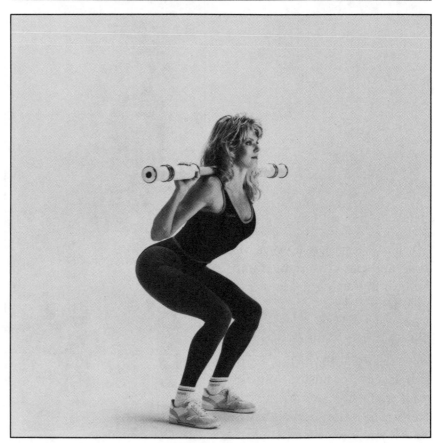

★Repeat this exercise 12 to 15 times★

Exercise 3.

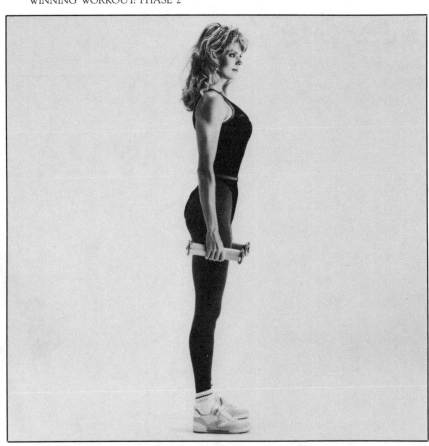

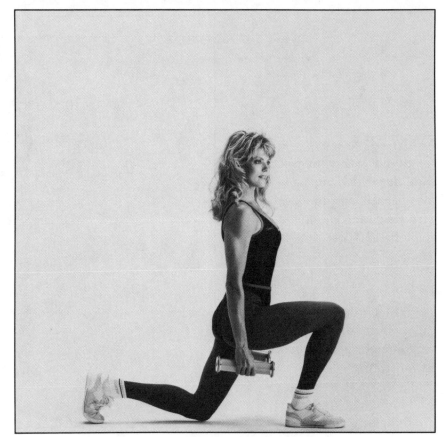

EXERCISE 3. Dumbbell Knee Lunges.

Holding a dumbbell in each hand, stand erect with your feet about 6″ to 10″ apart.

3A

Exhale as you step forward with one leg, bending your rear leg until your knee almost touches the floor. Keep your torso erect throughout this movement.

3B

Inhale as you step back and return to the starting position.

★Repeat this exercise eight to 12 times for each leg, alternating legs★

Exercise 4.

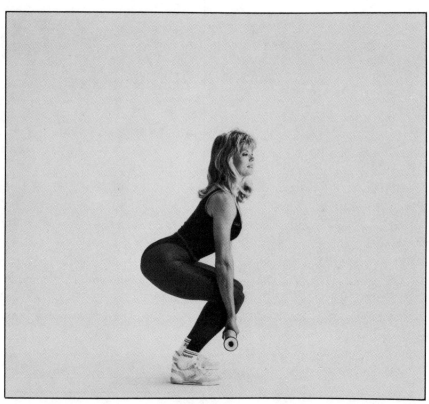

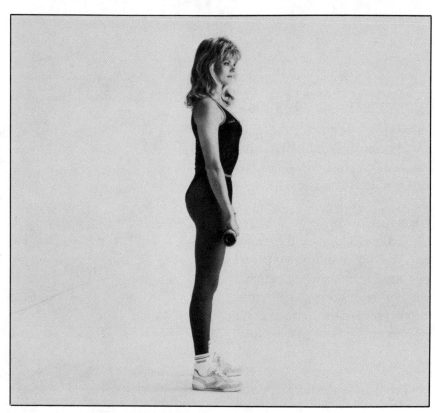

EXERCISE 4. Deadlifts.

Stand with your feet about shoulder-width apart. Grasp the barbell in an "over-grip," with your knuckles forward and your hands just outside your legs.

4A

Lower yourself to a squatting position, keeping your back straight and your head up as you inhale.

4B

Exhale as you stand

★Repeat this exercise 12 to 15 times★

Exercise 5.

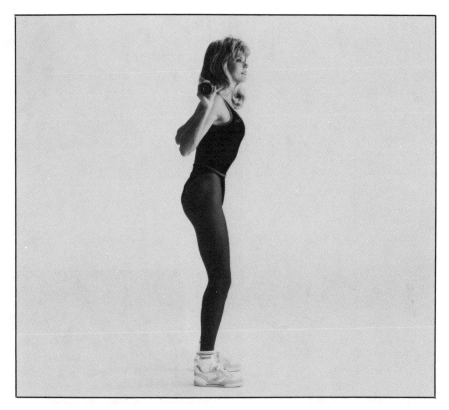

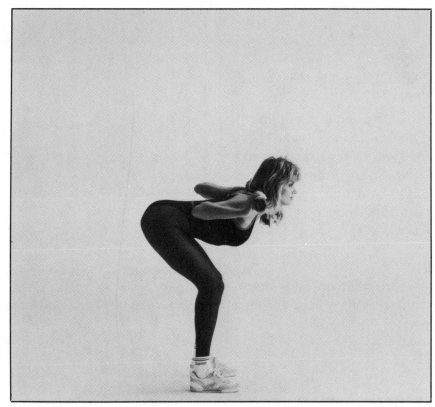

EXERCISE 5. Good-Mornings.
Position the barbell comfortably on your shoulders and bend your knees slightly.

5A
Inhale as you bend forward at the waist, keeping your back straight.

5B
Exhale as you return to the starting position.

★Repeat this exercise 12 to 15 times★

Exercise 6.

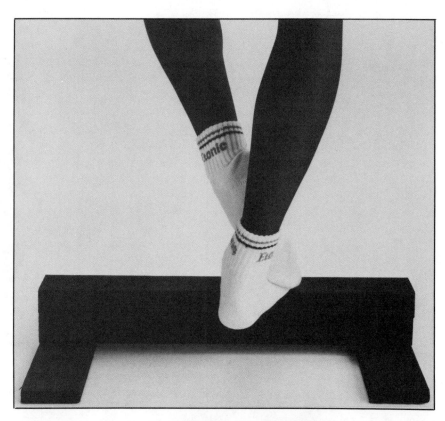

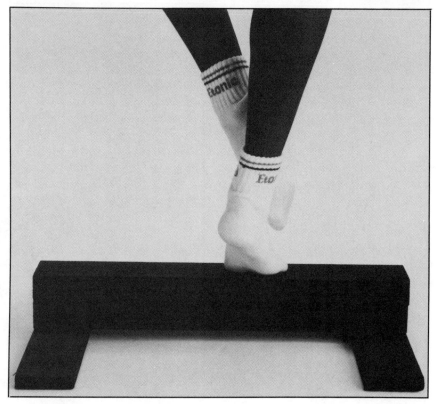

EXERCISE 6. One-legged Calf Raises.

Stand erect, holding a dumbbell in each hand. Place the ball of your right foot on a 2″ block, with your left foot on top of your right foot. Breathe normally throughout this exercise.

6A

Rise high on your tiptoes while keeping your right knee straight.

6B

Lower your right heel to the starting position.

★Repeat this exercise 15 to 20 times for each leg★

Exercise 7.

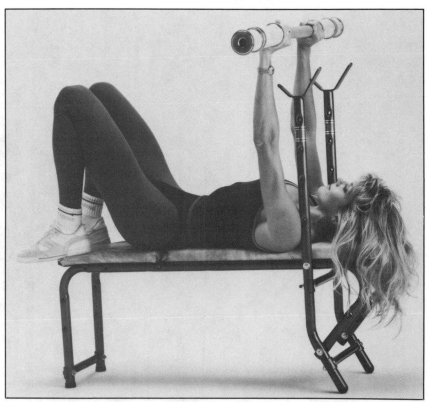

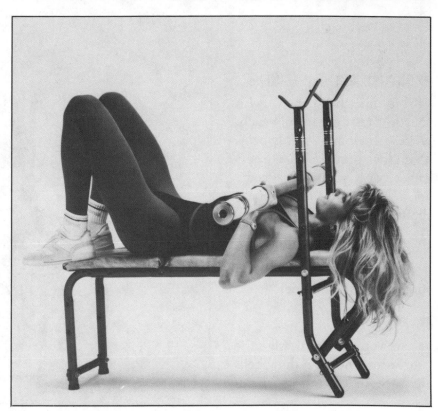

EXERCISE 7. Bench Presses.

Lie on the bench with your back flat and your feet resting either flat on the floor or on the bench. Remove the barbell from the support racks and hold it at arm's length overhead.

7A

Lower the barbell to your chest as you inhale.

7B

Press the barbell to the straight-arm position as you exhale.

★Repeat this exercise eight to 12 times★

Exercise 8.

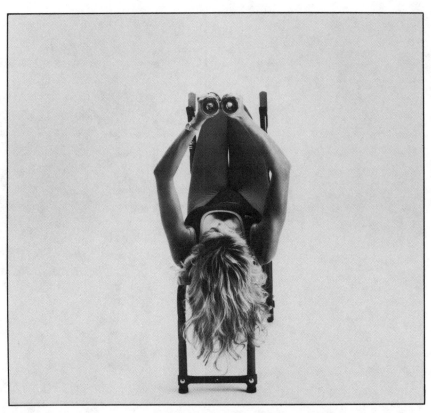

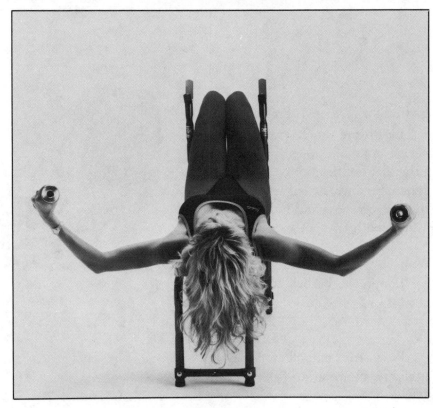

EXERCISE 8. Dumbbell Flies.

Lie on the bench, with your feet resting on the bench. With your elbows slightly bent, hold the dumbbell at arm's length, with your palms facing one another and the dumbbells about 2″ apart.

8A

Inhale deeply as you extend your arms to your sides.

8B

As you exhale, slowly raise your arms until the dumbbells are back in their original position.

★ Repeat this exercise eight to 12 times ★

Exercise 9.

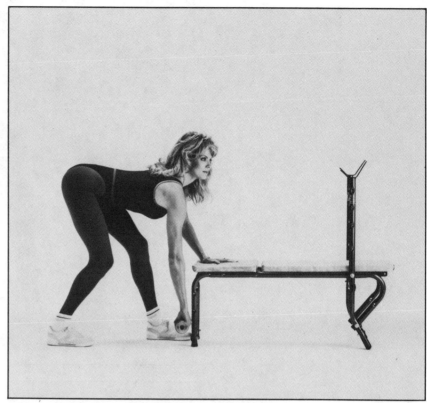

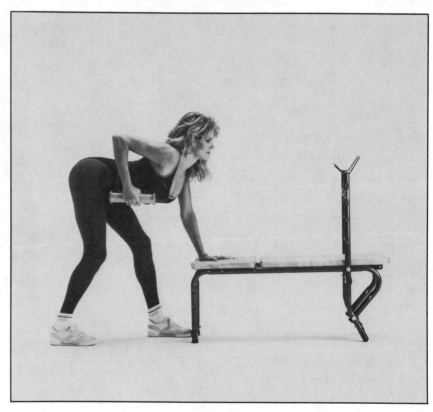

EXERCISE 9. One-Arm Dumbbell Bent Rows.

Stand at the end of the bench. Hold a dumbbell in your right hand and extend your right arm downward. Keep your knees bent and your back flat, place your left hand flat on the bench, and bend forward from your hips.

9A

Smoothly pull the dumbbell up to your chest, keeping your right elbow close to your body as you exhale.

9B

Lower the dumbbell to the starting position as you inhale.

★Repeat this exercise eight to 12 times for each arm★

Exercise 10.

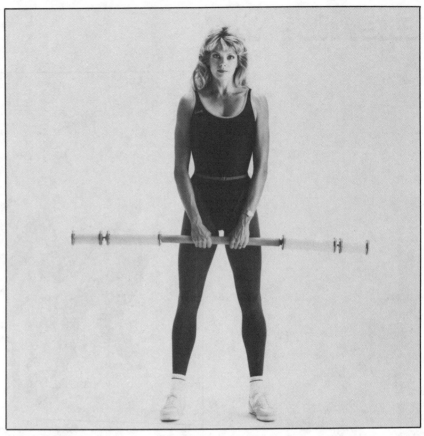

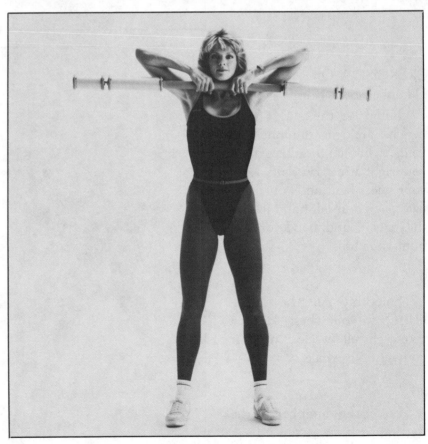

EXERCISE 10. Upright Rows.

Stand erect and hold the barbell in front of your thighs with your hands 4″ to 6″ apart.

10A

Exhale as you pull the barbell upward, keeping your elbows high until the barbell is under your chin.

10B

Inhale as you slowly lower the barbell to the starting position.

★Repeat this exercise eight to 12 times★

Exercise 11.

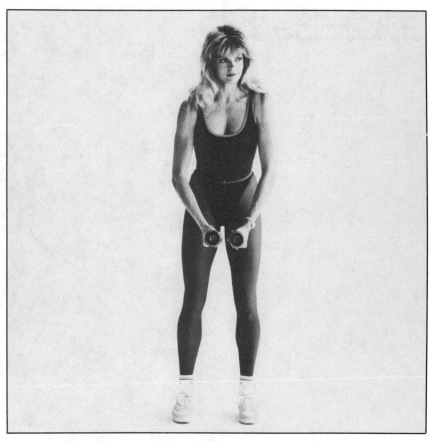

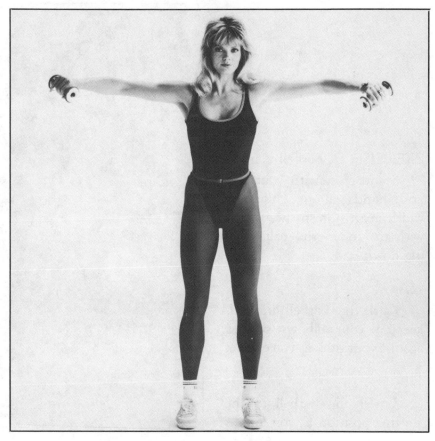

EXERCISE 11. Side Lateral Raises.

Stand erect with your feet about 12″ apart. Hold a dumb-bell in each hand, with your hands in front of your thighs and your arms slightly bent.

11A

Exhale as you raise your arms to your sides until they are shoulder-level.

11B

Inhale as you return to the starting position.

★Repeat this exercise eight to 12 times★

Exercise 12.

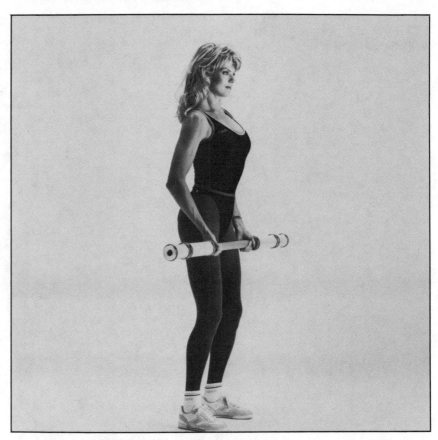

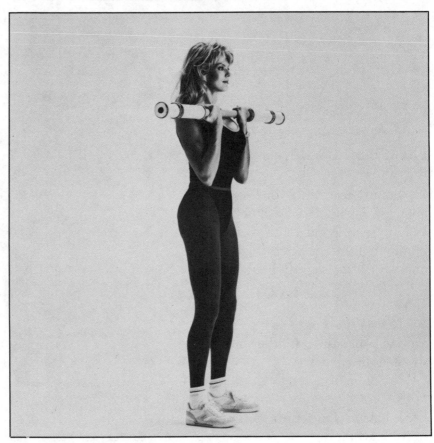

EXERCISE 12. Barbell Curls.

Stand erect with your feet and hands about shoulder-width apart. Grasp the barbell with an "under-grip," palms facing down.

12A

Curl the barbell upward, keeping your elbows pressed against your sides as you exhale.

12B

Lower the barbell to the starting position as you inhale.

★Repeat this exercise eight to 12 times★

Exercise 13.

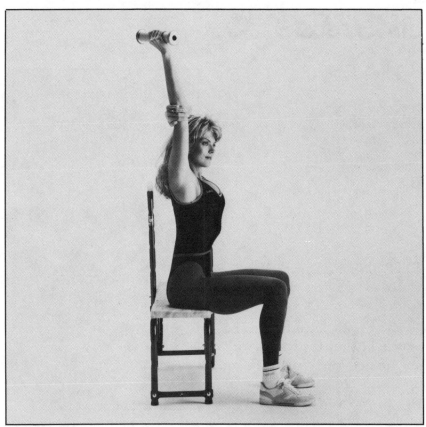

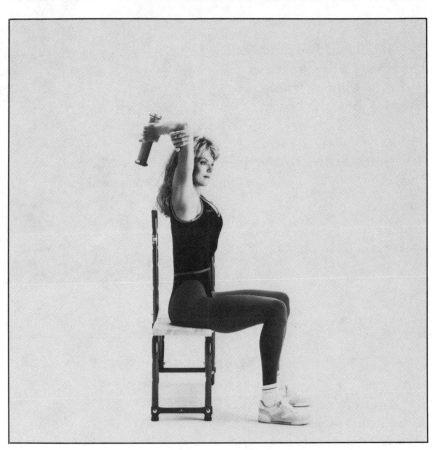

EXERCISE 13. Tricep Extensions.

Sit on the bench and hold a dumbbell at arm's length overhead. Reach across and grasp the elbow of your raised arm with your free hand.

13A

Inhale as you lower the dumbbell behind your head. Do not allow your elbow to move.

13B

Push the dumbbell back to the starting position as you inhale.

Repeat this exercise eight to 12 times for each arm

Exercise 14.

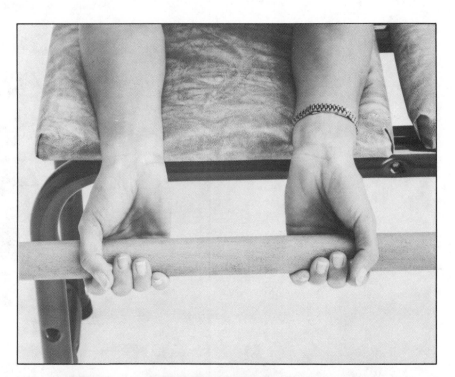

EXERCISE 14. Barbell Wrist Curls and Reverse Wrist Curls.

Rest both forearms on the bench, holding the barbell with an "under-grip," palms facing up. Bend both wrists down as far as you can. Breathe normally throughout this exercise.

14A

Grip the barbell firmly and bend both wrists up as far as you can, without letting your forearms leave the bench.

14B

Return to the starting position.

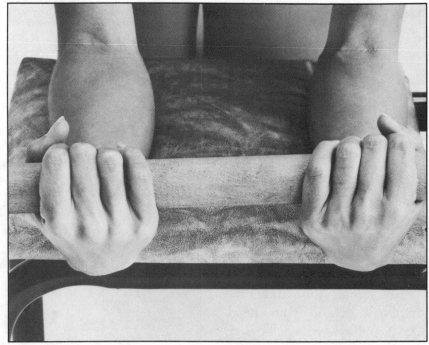

★Repeat this exercise 15 to 20 times★

Reverse Wrist Curls are performed the same way, except that an "over-grip" (palms facing down) is used.

★Repeat Reverse Wrist Curls 15 to 20 times★

Exercise 15.

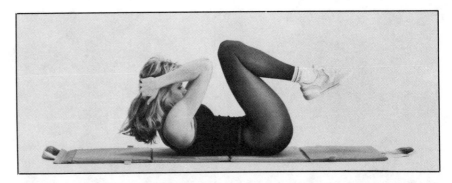

EXERCISE 15. Four-Part Sit-Up Routine.

Lie on your back with your knees bent and your feet off the floor. Clasp your hands behind your head. Don't hold your breath—breathe comfortably throughout this exercise.

15A

Raise your head, shoulders, and upper back and bring your elbows up to your knees.

15B

Straighten your legs while reaching your hands toward your ankles.

15C

Return to elbow-knee position.

15D

Spread your legs in a V and reach through them with your arms.

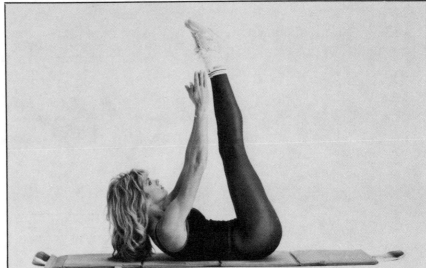

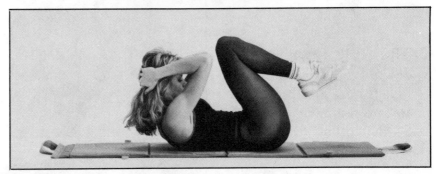

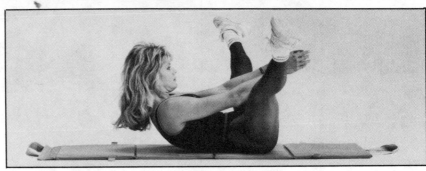

★Repeat this exercise 10 times★

Exercise 16.

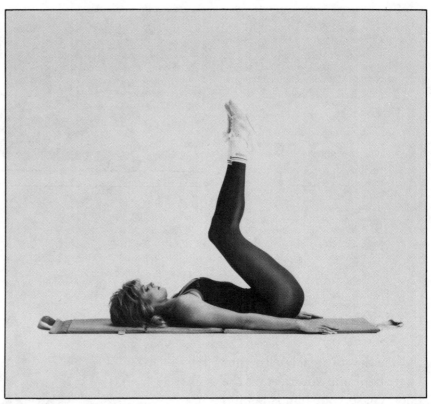

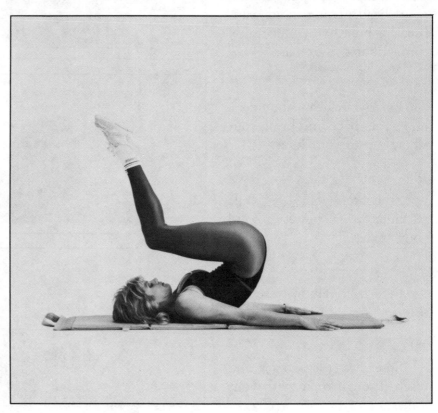

EXERCISE 16. Reverse Curl-Ups.

Lie flat on your back, with your arms resting at your sides and your palms flat on the floor.

16A

With slightly bent knees, exhale as you raise your legs, buttocks, and lower back toward your chest.

16B

Slowly return to the starting position as you inhale.

★Repeat this exercise 10 times★

Exercise 17.

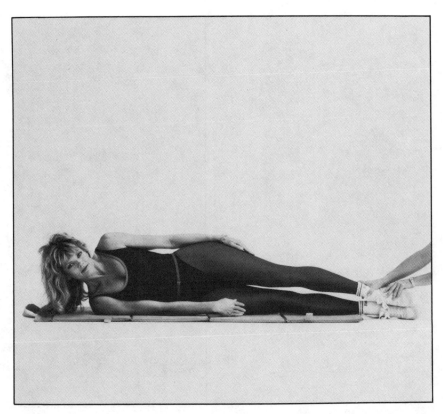

EXERCISE 17. Floor Side Bends.

Lie on your left side. Have someone hold your feet down, or brace them under the bottom rung of a wall bar. Don't hold your breath—breathe comfortably throughout this exercise.

17A

Keeping your arms at your sides, lift your head and shoulders as much as you can by bending at the waist.

17B

Return to floor.

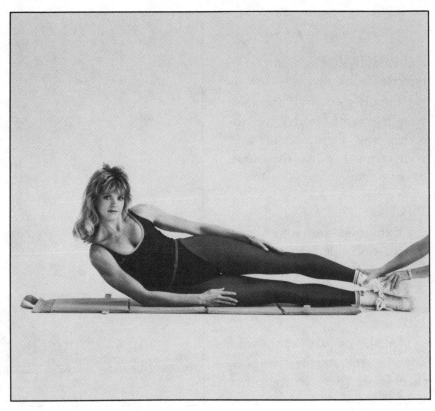

★Repeat this exercise 20 to 30 times on each side★

Exercise 18.

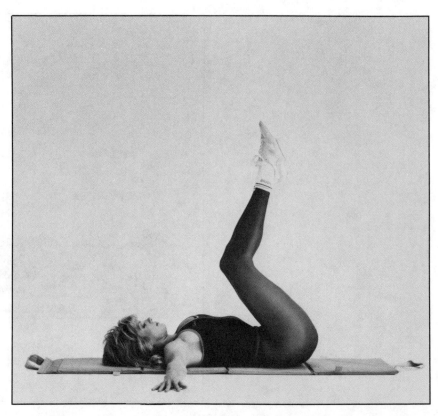

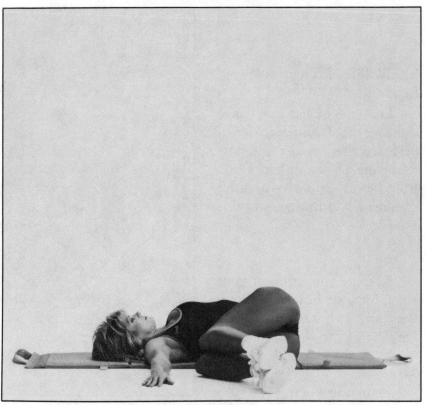

EXERCISE 18. Beginning Reverse Trunk Twists.

Lie on your back and raise your legs, with your knees together and slightly bent, and your arms out to the sides, palms down.

18A

Exhale as you lower your legs to one side, keeping your knees together and your shoulders and arms flat on the floor.

18B

Inhale as you raise your knees to the starting position, then lower them to the other side.

★ Repeat this exercise 20 to 30 times for each side, alternating sides ★

Now do the Cool-Down and Stretch described in Chapter 9.

CHAPTER EIGHT

Winning Workout: Phase 3

Good for you! You've now reached the most advanced phase of your program. There's no question that at this point you've already made enormous improvements in your level of strength, muscle endurance, and overall conditioning. If you haven't already started to see a big difference in the way you look, you will over the next four weeks, particularly if you've been following my advice and getting plenty of aerobic exercise along with your weight-training workouts. You should have no trouble sticking to your exercise routine by now, and I hope that by the time you finish Phase 3, you'll be so hooked on working out that you'll continue to use the program to maintain the new, improved you.

Once again, I've added some new exercises and a few new twists to some of the ones you already know. Every week you'll do three sets of reps, the maximum even for the most serious weight trainers, but for the last two weeks, I want you to increase the amount of weight you lift. Remember, do this in small increments, testing first to make sure you haven't added too much weight all at once.

I think you're going to find Phase 3 challenging and a lot of fun. Continue to polish your exercise form, and try to develop even greater sensitivity to your body's responses throughout this phase. At this level, you can begin to focus on the finer points of your technique, and on the subtle changes in your body awareness. Phase 3 is a challenge, but you're ready for it. I'm proud of you, and you should be proud of you, too!

Winning Workout / Phase 3

EXERCISE	REPETITIONS	THIGHS	BUTTOCKS	HIPS	QUADS	LOWER BACK	HAM-STRINGS	CALVES
1. Step-Ups with barbell	15 for each leg	X	X	X				X
2. Barbell squats	12 to 15	X	X	X	X	X		
3. Barbell squats with feet turned in	12 to 15	X	X	X		X		
4. Barbell squats with feet turned out	12 to 15	X	X	X		X		
5. Straight-leg barbell lunges	12 to 15		X		X		X	
6. Deadlifts	12 to 15						X	
7., 8., 9. Calf raises with dumbbells, 3 positions	12 to 15							X
10. Push-ups	15 to 20							
11. Barbell bench presses	8 to 12							
12. Dumbbell Flies	8 to 12							
13. Seated barbell presses behind neck	8 to 12							
14. Barbell bent rows	8 to 12							
15. Cross bench pullovers	8 to 12							
16. Barbell upright rows	8 to 12							
17. Military presses	8 to 12							
18. Side lateral dumbbell raises	8 to 12							
19., 20. Barbell curls, 2 positions	8 to 12							
21. Alternate dumbbell curls	8 to 12							
22. Tricep extensions with barbell	8 to 12							
23. Underhand and overhand wrist curls with barbell	15 to 20							
24. 4-Part sit-up routine	10 cycles							
25. Floor side bends	40 to 50 each side							
26. Reverse curl-ups	40 to 50							
27. Advanced reverse trunk twists	40 to 50 each side							

*Weeks 1 through 4: 3 sets

PECTORALS	DELTOIDS	TRICEPS	LATS	BICEPS	SPINAL ERECTORS	TRAPEZIUS	FOREARMS	ABDOM-INALS	INTERNAL OBLIQUE	EXTERNAL OBLIQUE	WAIST
					X						
X		X									
X	X	X									
X	X										
	X	X									
			X	X	X	X					
X			X								
	X			X		X					
	X	X									
	X					X					
				X							
				X							
		X									
							X				
								X			
									X	X	X
											X
									X	X	X

Summary of Repetitions / Phase 3

	Week 9	Week 10	Week 11	Week 12	
	3 sets	3 sets	3 sets	3 sets	
			add weight	add weight	
UPPER BODY	8 to 10	10 to 12	10 to 12	10 to 12	Repetitions
LOWER BODY	12 to 13	13 to 15	13 to 15	13 to 15	Repetitions
ABDOMINALS AND OBLIQUES	20 to 30	20 to 30	30 to 40	30 to 40	Repetitions

Exercise 1.

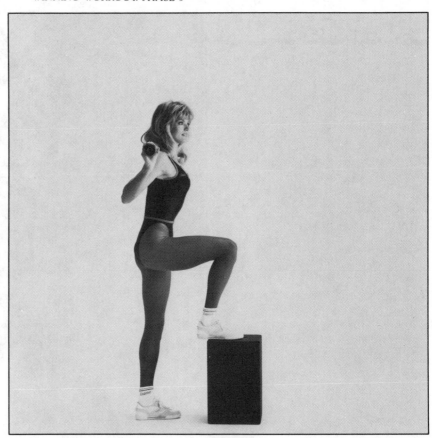

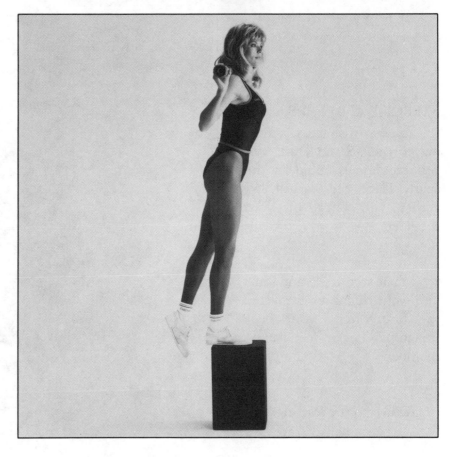

EXERCISE 1. Step-Ups with Barbell.

Position the barbell comfortably on your shoulders.

1A

Place your right foot flat on the box.

1B

Step up onto the box as you exhale, without pushing off with your left leg.

1C

Return to the starting position as you inhale.

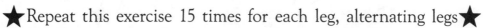

★Repeat this exercise 15 times for each leg, alternating legs★

113

Exercise 2.

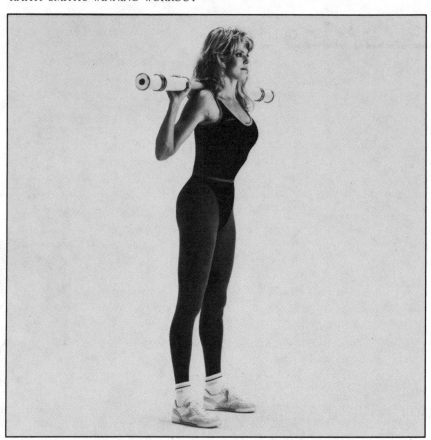

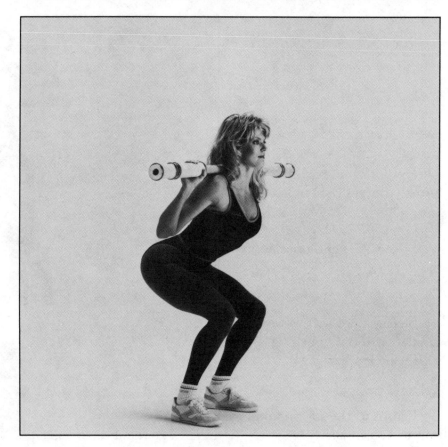

EXERCISE 2. Barbell Squats.

You may wish to use a training partner. Stand erect with your feet about shoulder-width apart. Place the barbell low across the back of your shoulders.

2A

Inhale vigorously and squat until your thighs are parallel to the floor. Keep your back straight and your feet flat on the floor.

2B

Return to the starting position as you inhale.

★Repeat this exercise 12 to 15 times★

Exercise 3.

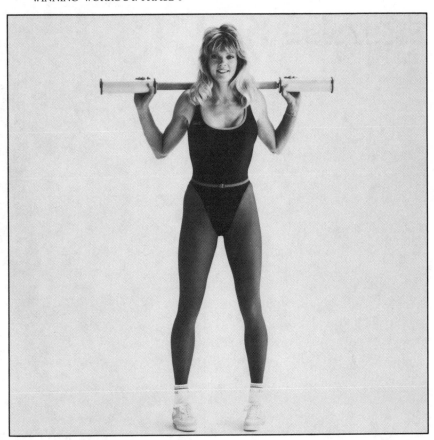

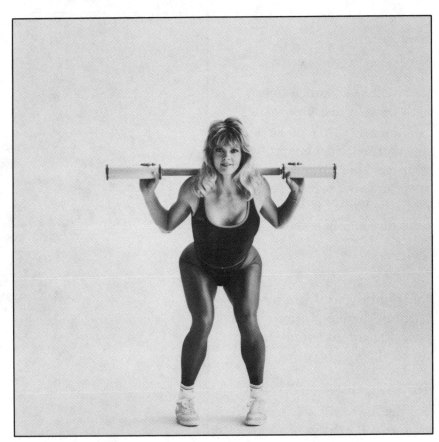

EXERCISE 3. Barbell Squats with Feet Turned In.

You may wish to use a training partner. Stand erect with your feet about shoulder-width apart and your toes turned in. Place the barbell low across the back of your shoulders.

3A

As you inhale vigorously, squat until your thighs are parallel to the floor. Keep your back straight and your feet flat on the floor.

3B

Return to the starting position as you exhale.

★Repeat this exercise 12 to 15 times★

Exercise 4.

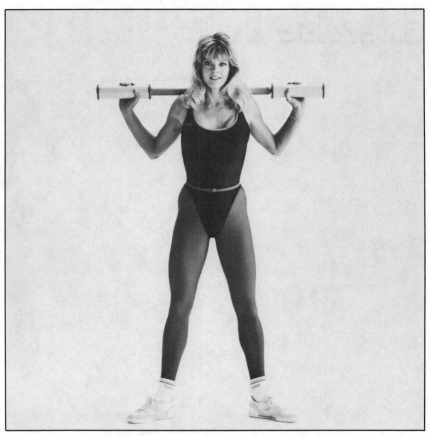

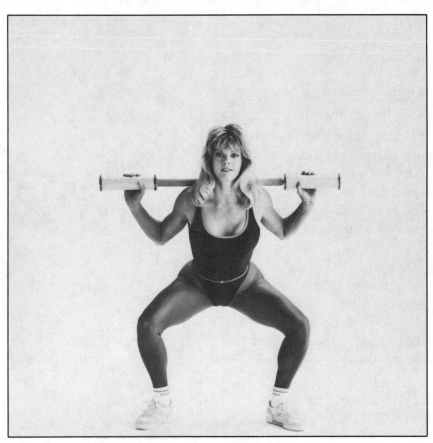

EXERCISE 4. Barbell Squats with Feet Turned Out.

You may wish to use a training partner. Stand erect with your feet about shoulder-width apart and your toes turned out. Place the barbell low across the back of your shoulders.

4A

As you inhale vigorously, squat until your thighs are parallel to the floor. Keep your back straight and your feet flat on the floor.

4B

Return to the starting position as you exhale.

★Repeat this exercise 12 to 15 times★

Exercise 5.

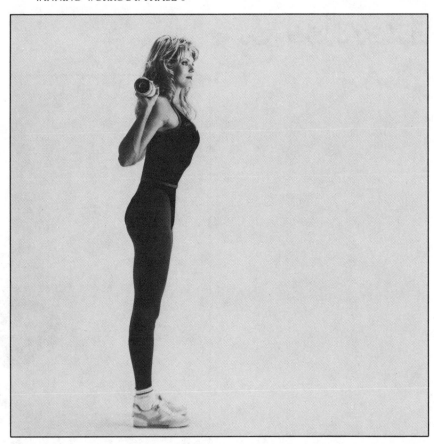

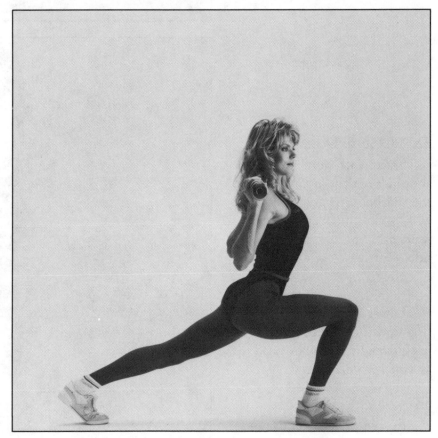

EXERCISE 5. Straight-Leg Barbell Lunges.

Stand erect with the barbell resting across your shoulders behind your neck and your feet about 12″ apart.

5A

Exhale as you step forward as far as possible with your right foot, keeping your left leg straight and your left foot in place.

5B

Return to the starting position as you inhale.

★Repeat this exercise 12 to 15 times for each leg, alternating legs★

Exercise 6.

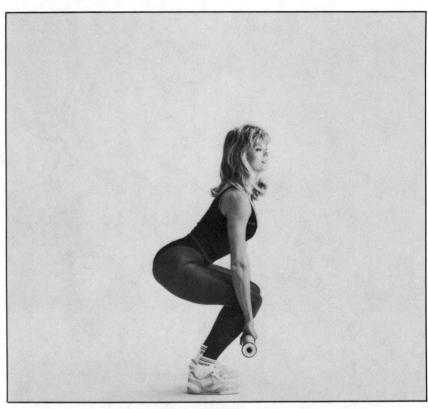

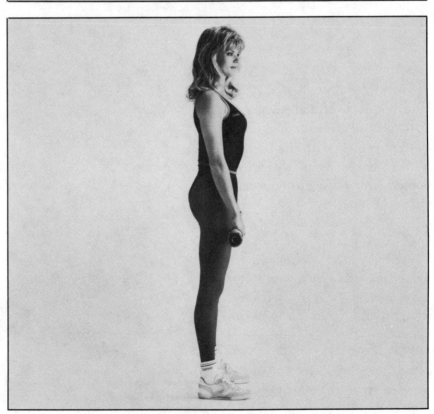

EXERCISE 6. Deadlifts.

Stand with your feet about shoulder-width apart. Grasp the barbell in an "over-grip," with your knuckles facing forward and your hands just outside your legs.

6A

Lower yourself to a squatting position, keeping your back straight and your head up as you inhale.

6B

Exhale as you stand

★ Repeat this exercise 12 to 15 times ★

Exercise 7.

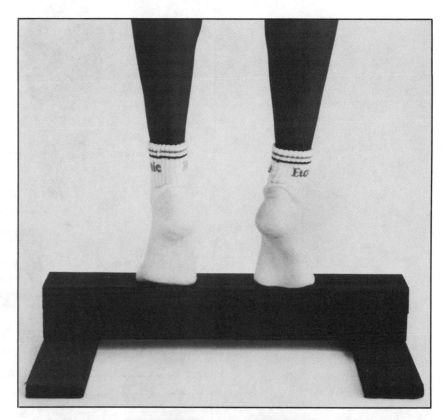

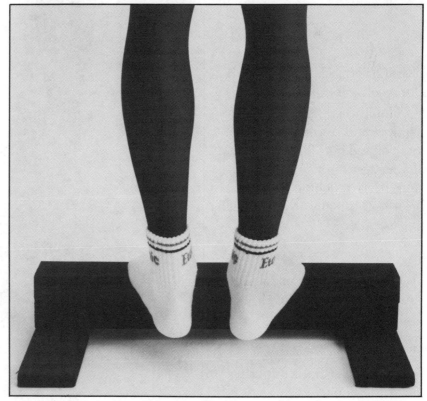

EXERCISE 7. Calf Raises with Dumbbells.

Holding a dumbbell in each hand, stand erect with your feet parallel. Place the balls of your feet on a 2″ block, with your heels touching the floor. Breathe normally throughout this exercise.

7A

Rise high on your tiptoes while keeping your knees straight.

7B

Lower your heels until they touch the floor.

★Repeat this exercise 12 to 15 times★

Exercise 8.

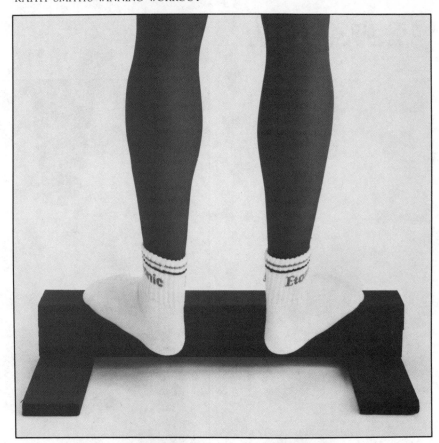

EXERCISE 8. Calf Raises with Dumbbells, Toes Pointed Out.

Holding a dumbbell in each hand, stand erect with your toes pointed out. Place the balls of your feet on a 2″ block with your heels touching the floor. Breathe normally throughout this exercise.

8A

Rise high on your tiptoes while keeping your knees straight.

8B

Lower your heels until they touch the floor.

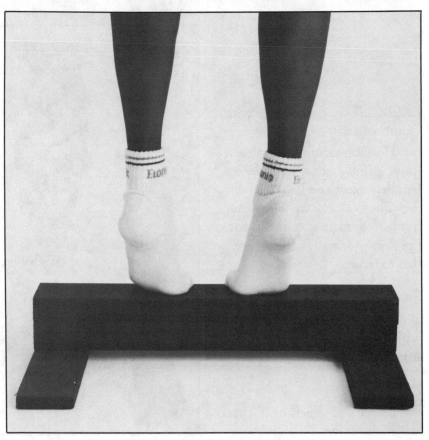

★ Repeat this exercise 12 to 15 times ★

Exercise 9.

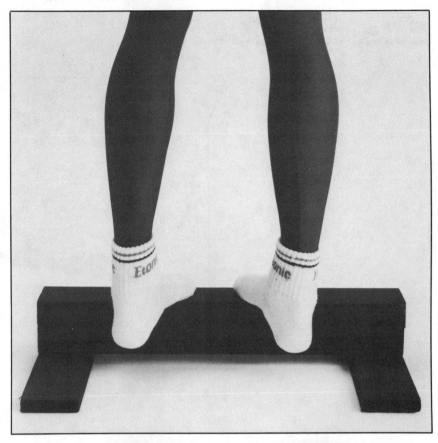

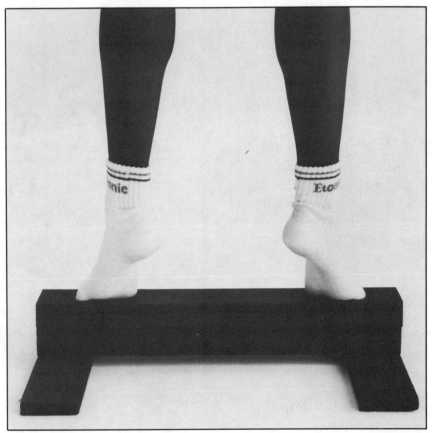

EXERCISE 9. Calf Raises with Dumbbells, Toes Pointed In.

Holding a dumbbell in each hand, stand erect with your toes pointed in. Place the balls of your feet on a 2″ block with your heels touching the floor. Breathe normally throughout this exercise.

9A

Rise high on your tiptoes while keeping your knees straight.

9B

Lower your heels until they touch the floor.

★ Repeat this exercise 12 to 15 times ★

Exercise 10.

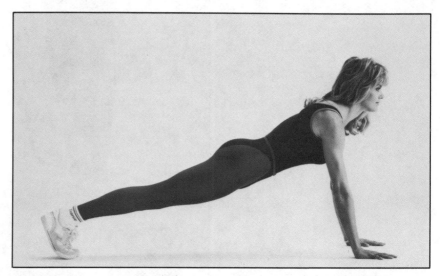

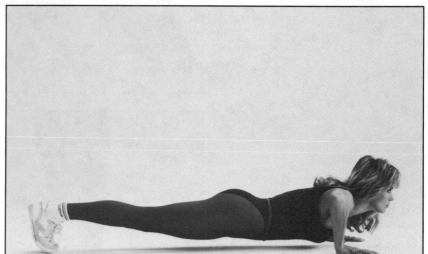

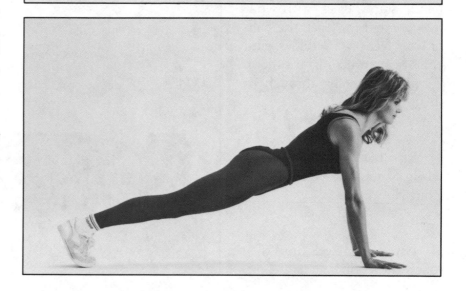

EXERCISE 10. Push-Ups.

Kneel on the floor and assume a "push-up" position, holding your body straight and your hands shoulder-width apart.

10A

Inhale as you lower yourself as low as possible, but keep your body straight from head to foot.

10B

Return to the starting position as you exhale.

★Repeat this exercise 15 to 20 times★

Exercise 11

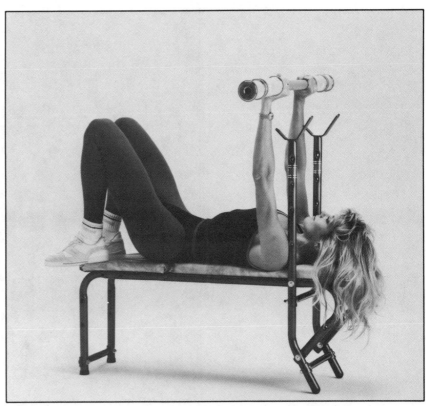

EXERCISE 11. Barbell Bench Presses.

You may wish to use a training partner. Lie on the bench with your back flat and your feet resting either flat on the floor or on the bench. Remove the barbell from the support racks, and hold it overhead at arm's length.

11A

Lower the barbell to your chest as you inhale.

11B

Press the barbell to the straight-arm position as you inhale.

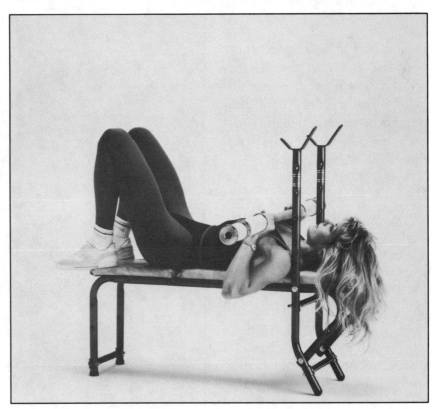

★Repeat this exercise 12 to 15 times★

Exercise 12.

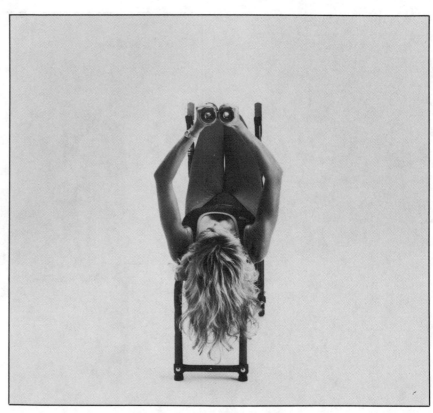

EXERCISE 12. Dumbbell Flies.

Lie on the bench with your back flat and your feet resting on the bench. With your elbows slightly bent, hold the dumbbells at arm's length with your palms facing and the dumbbells about 2″ apart.

12A

With your arms slightly bent, lower the dumbbells out to the sides as far as possible as you inhale deeply. Do not straighten your arms.

12B

As you exhale, slowly raise your arms until the dumbbells are back in their original position, 2″ apart.

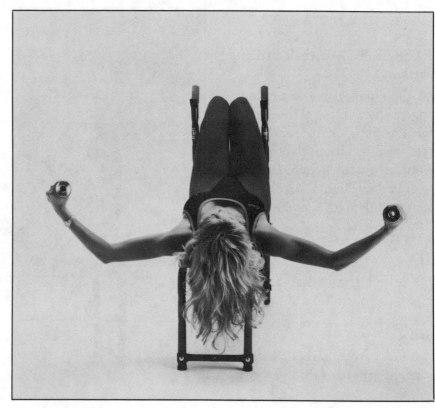

★ Repeat this exercise eight to 12 times ★

Exercise 13.

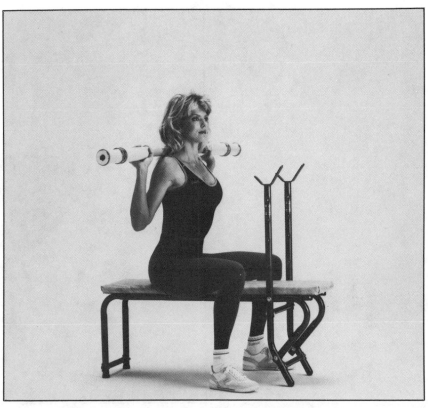

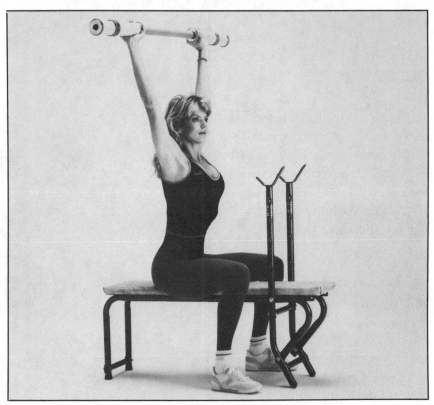

EXERCISE 13. Seated Barbell Presses Behind the Neck.

You may wish to use a training partner. Sitting astride the bench, hold the barbell across your shoulders behind your neck. Use a wide grip.

13A

Exhale as you press the barbell to arm's length overhead.

13B

Return to the starting position as you inhale.

★Repeat this exercise eight to 12 times★

Exercise 14.

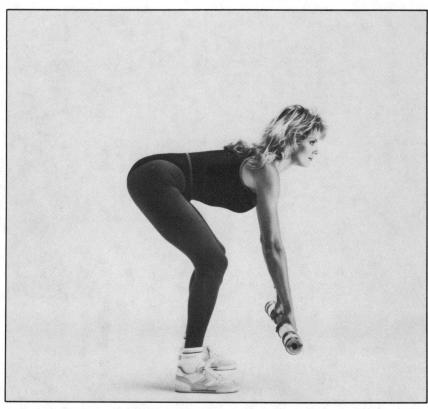

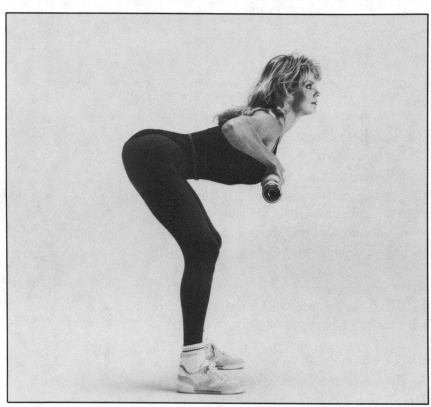

EXERCISE 14. Barbell Bent Rows.

With your arms extended down and your hands shoulder-width apart, grasp the barbell with an "over-grip," knuckles facing out. Lean forward from your hips, keeping your back flat and bending both legs.

14A

As you exhale, pull the barbell up until it touches your chest.

14B

Lower the barbell to the starting position as you inhale.

★ Repeat this exercise eight to 12 times ★

Exercise 15.

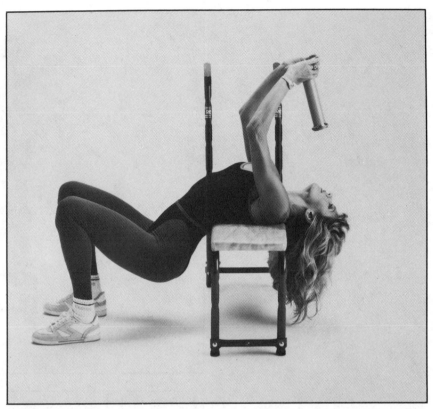

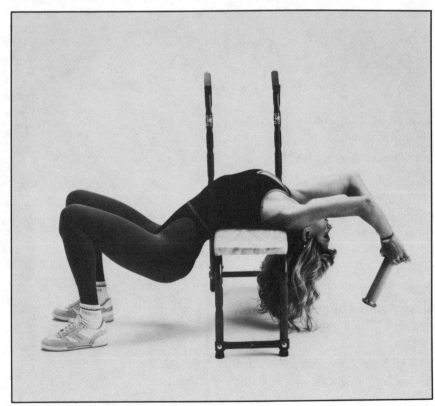

EXERCISE 15. Cross-Bench Pullovers.

Lie across the bench with your shoulders resting on the bench and with your hips lower than the bench. Place your feet apart, flat on the floor. Interlace your fingers around the end of one dumbbell, and extend both arms.

15A

Keeping your feet flat on the floor, inhale and lower the dumbbell to the rear with your arms slightly bent.

15B

Return to the starting position as you exhale.

★Repeat this exercise eight to 12 times★

Exercise 16.

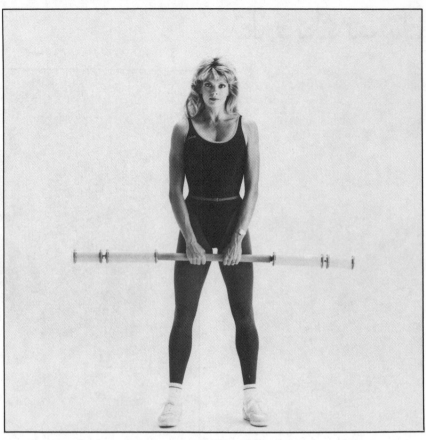

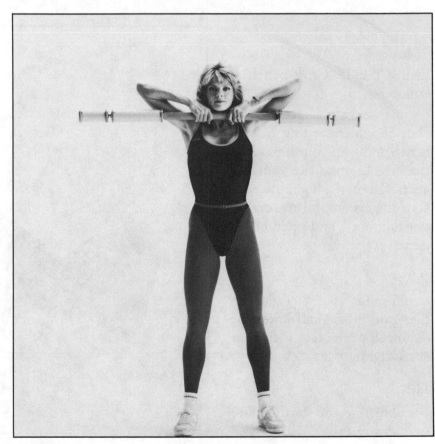

EXERCISE 16. Barbell Upright Rows.

Stand erect, holding the barbell in front of your thighs, with your hands 4″ to 6″ apart.

16A

Exhale as you pull the barbell upward, keeping your elbows high until the barbell is under your chin.

16B

Inhale as you return smoothly and slowly to the starting position.

★Repeat this exercise eight to 12 times★

Exercise 17.

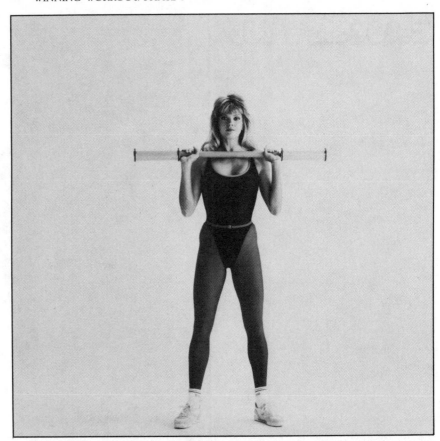

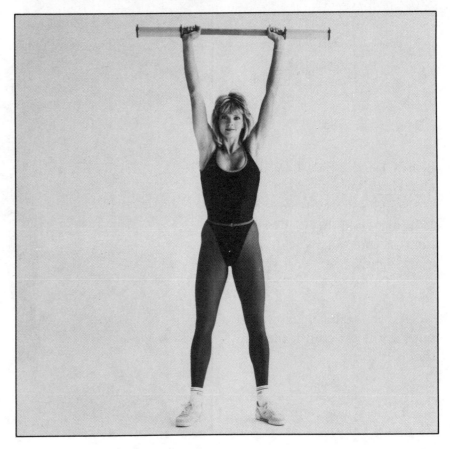

EXERCISE 17. Military Presses.

Position the barbell at your shoulders, hands facing out.

17A

Keeping your back and legs straight, exhale as you press the barbell upward until your arms are extended overhead.

17B

Lower to the starting position as you inhale.

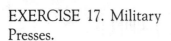★Repeat this exercise eight to 12 times★

Exercise 18.

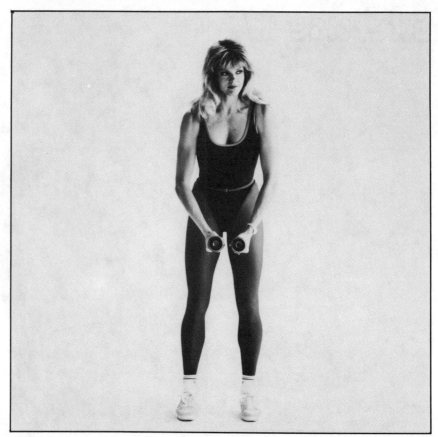

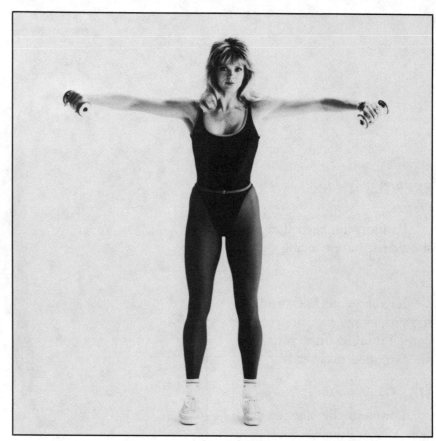

EXERCISE 18. Side Lateral Dumbbell Raises.

Stand erect with your feet 12" apart. Hold the dumbbell in front of your thighs with your arms slightly bent.

18A

As you exhale, raise your arms to the sides until they are shoulder-level.

18B

Inhale as you return to the starting position.

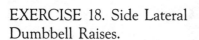 Repeat this exercise eight to 12 times ★

Exercise 19.

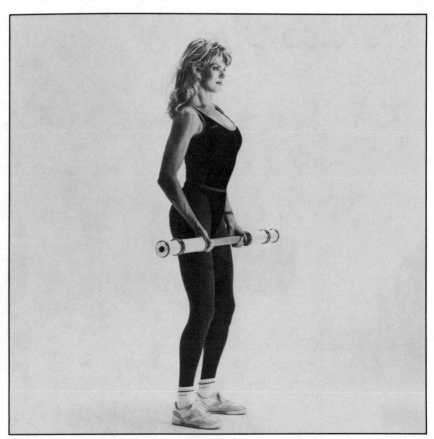

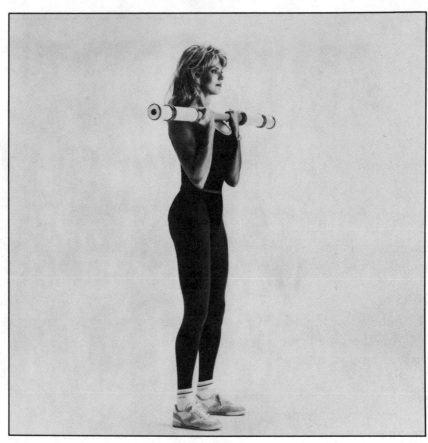

EXERCISE 19. Barbell Curls.

Stand erect with your feet about shoulder-width apart. Grasp the barbell with an "under-grip," palms facing out, hands shoulder-width apart.

19A

Exhale as you curl the barbell up, keeping your elbows pressed against your sides.

19B

Inhale as you return to the starting position.

★ Repeat this exercise 10 to 15 times ★

Exercise 20.

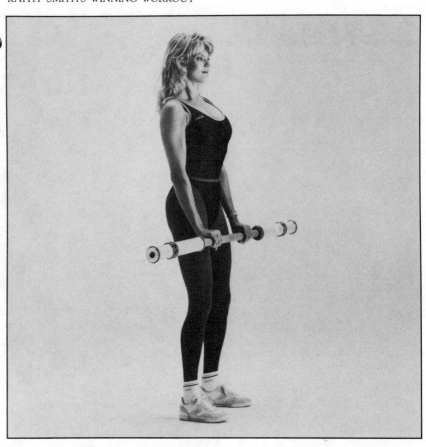

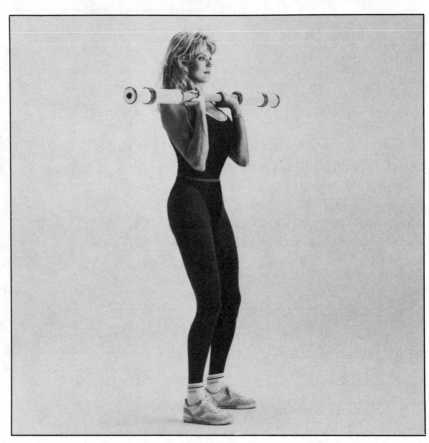

EXERCISE 20. Reverse Barbell Curls.

This exercise is performed the same as Barbell Curls, except that an "over-grip" (palms facing down) is used.

20A

Exhale as you curl the barbell up, keeping your elbows pressed against your sides.

20B

Inhale as you return to the starting position.

★ Repeat this exercise eight to 12 times ★

Exercise 21.

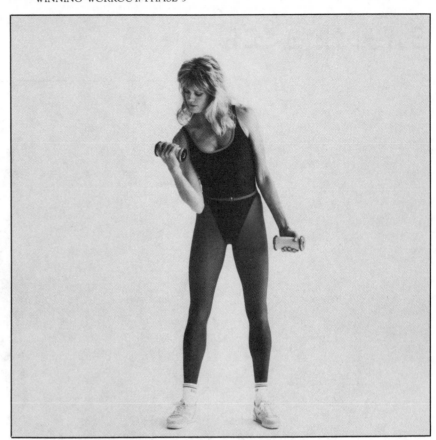

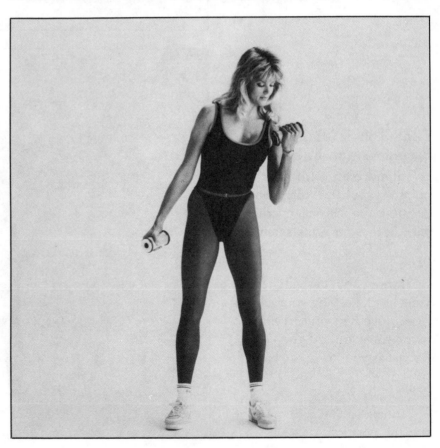

EXERCISE 21. Alternate Dumbbell Curls.

Stand with your feet about 12″ apart. Grasp the dumbbells, one in each hand, with your palms forward and your arms extended straight down.

21A

Curl one dumbbell up until it touches your shoulder as you exhale. Then lower the dumbbell as you inhale.

21B

Curl the other dumbbell up to your other shoulder as you exhale. Then lower the dumbbell as you inhale.

★Repeat this exercise eight to 12 times for each arm, alternating arms★

Exercise 22.

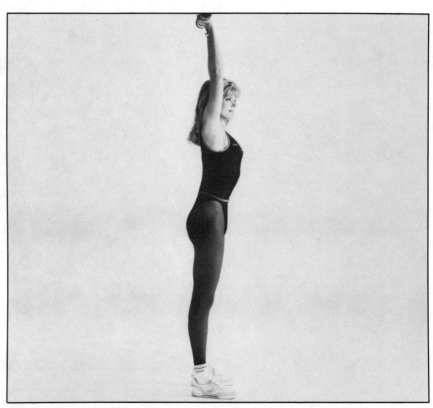

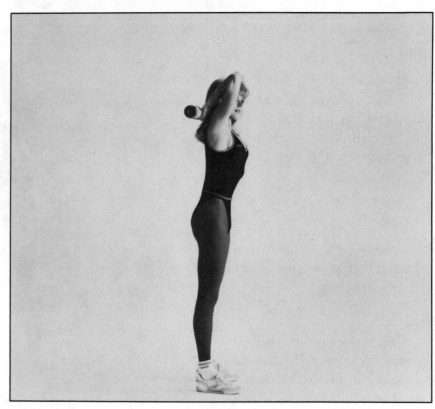

EXERCISE 22. Tricep Extensions with Barbell.

Stand erect with your feet about shoulder-width apart. Position the barbell overhead, with both your arms extended.

22A

Lower the barbell behind your head, keeping your elbows close together and trying to point them toward the ceiling. Exhale as you lower the barbell.

22B

Inhale as you return to the starting position.

★Repeat this exercise eight to 12 times★

Exercise 23.

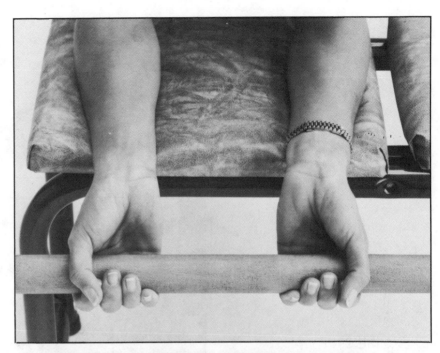

EXERCISE 23. Underhand and Overhand Wrist Curls with Barbell.

For an Underhand Wrist Curl, rest both your forearms along the top of the bench, holding the barbells with an "under-grip," palms facing up. Bend both your wrists down as far as you can. Breathe normally throughout this exercise.

23A

Grip the barbell firmly and bend both your wrists up as far as you can, without letting your forearms leave the bench. Return to the starting position.

23B

Overhand Wrist Curls are performed the same as Underhand Wrist Curls, except that an "over-grip" (palms facing down) is used.

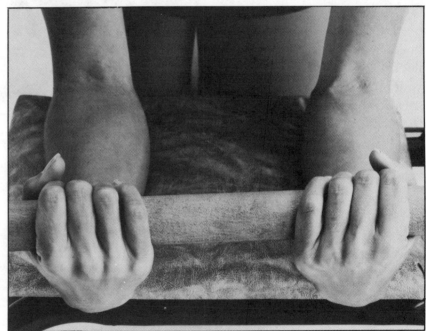

★Repeat this exercise 15 to 20 times★

★Repeat Overhand Wrist Curls 15 to 20 times★

135

Exercise 24.

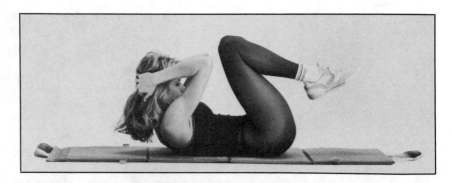

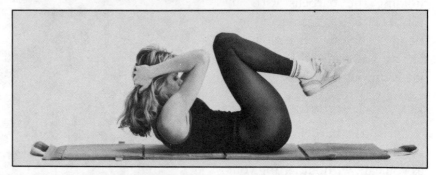

EXERCISE 24. Four-Part Sit-Up Routine.

Lie on your back with your knees bent and your feet off the floor. Clasp your hands behind your head. Don't hold your breath—breathe comfortably throughout this exercise.

24A

Bring your elbows up to your knees.

24B

Straighten your legs as you reach your hands up to your ankles.

24C

Return to elbows-to-knees position.

24D

Spread your legs in a V and reach through them with your arms.

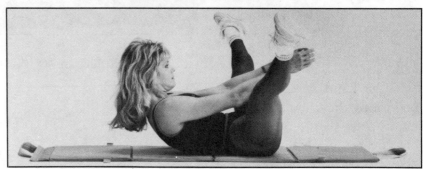

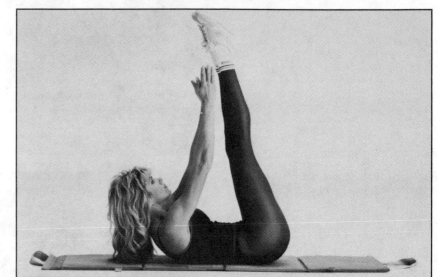

★Repeat this exercise 10 times★

Exercise 25.

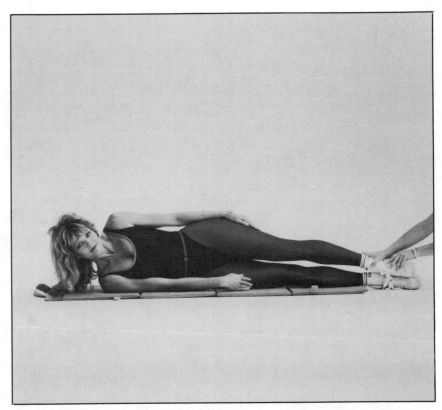

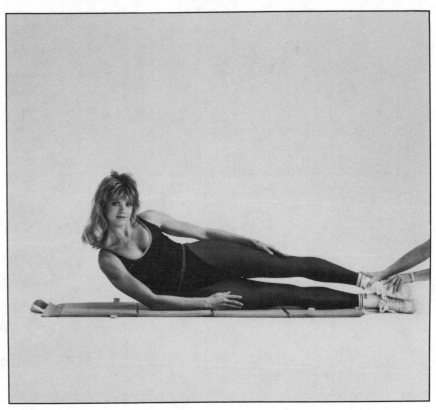

EXERCISE 25. Floor Side Bends.

Lie on your left side. Have someone hold your feet down, or place them under the bottom rung of a wall bar. Don't hold your breath—breathe comfortably throughout this exercise.

25A

Keep your arms at your sides and lift your head and shoulders as much as you can by bending at your waist.

25B

Return to the starting position.

★Repeat this exercise 40 to 50 times for each side★

Exercise 26.

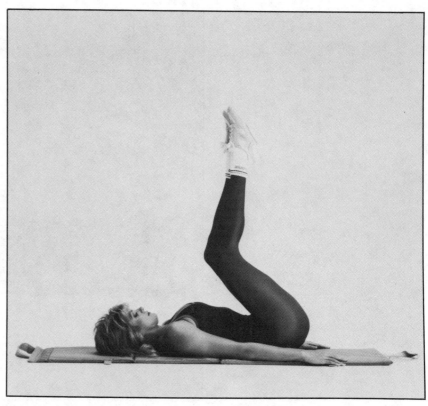

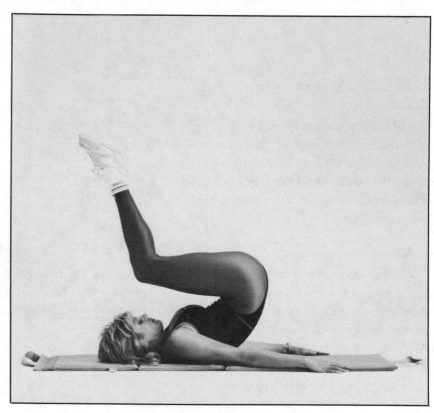

EXERCISE 26. Reverse Curl-Ups.

Lie flat on your back with your arms at your sides and your palms flat on the floor.

26A

With your knees slightly bent, raise your legs, buttocks, and lower back up toward your chest as you exhale.

26B

Return to the starting position as you inhale.

★Repeat this exercise 40 to 50 times★

Exercise 27.

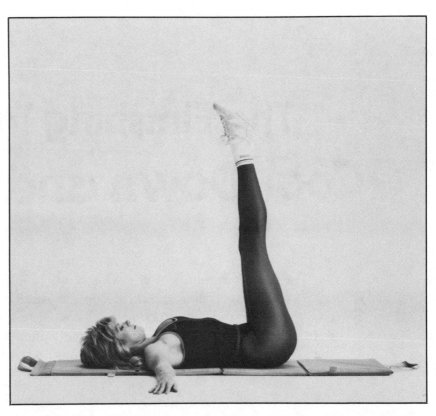

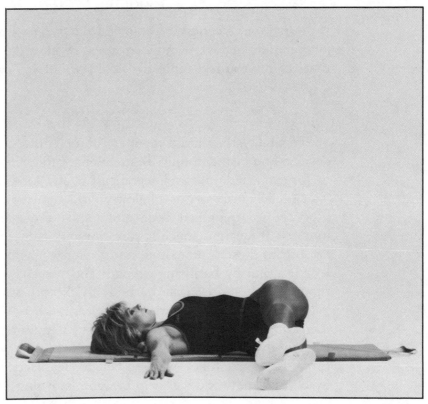

EXERCISE 27. Advanced Reverse Trunk Twists.

Lie on your back with your legs raised at a 90° angle, and your arms out to the sides, palms down.

27A

As you exhale, lower your legs to one side and touch the floor, keeping your shoulders and arms flat on the floor.

27B

Raise your legs as you inhale, and then lower them to the other side as you exhale.

★Repeat this exercise 40 to 50 times for each side, alternating sides★

Now do the Cool-Down and Stretch described in Chapter 9.

CHAPTER NINE

The Finishing Touch: Cool-Down and Stretch

The cool-down phase of your workout is as important as the warm-up, even though it takes you in the opposite direction. Now you need to give your heart and circulatory system a chance to slow gradually to their normal operating level. If you stop suddenly after strenuous exercise, all the extra blood that's pumping through your body will pool in your lower extremities, leaving you feeling weak, dizzy, and possibly a bit faint.

Cooling Down

After you've completed your last set of reps, walk around the room for a minute or two, swing your arms, or lift a light weight a few extra times before you segue into the final stage of your workout, the stretch.

Stretching

Flexibility, the third component of total fitness, is something you can develop and maintain only by stretching. Stretching isn't something you do for extra credit. It's an integral part of any good exercise program, and it's especially necessary as a follow-up to weight training. This is because, in order to strengthen your muscles, you've been contracting them intensely throughout much of your workout. Now you need to relax every last one of those contractions, and stretch your muscles out to their full length again. By balancing strength and stretch, you'll develop muscles that are long and lean, and a body that's both strong and graceful.

Now, rather than during your warm-up, is the time to work on increasing your flexibility. After weight training, your muscles are thoroughly warm and, like warm rubber or clay, they're at their most pliable. A good stretch now will also help to clear lactic acid and other toxins from your body, and will help prevent "morning-after" muscle soreness.

You'll still want to keep your movements gentle and flowing, and to avoid any violent bouncing. The one inviolable rule is: *Never try to force a stretch, only to coax it.* Flexibility is largely inherited, and although you can improve your flexibility, you'll have to work within your given limits. It's utterly pointless, as well as dangerous, to try to compete with someone who can stretch farther than you can. It's also counterproductive. If you try to force a stretch, your muscles will rebel by contracting and becoming more intractable than ever. By contrast, stretching gently, preferably on a nice, soothing exhale, relaxes and lengthens your muscles naturally; it's a way of telling them that everything is fine and that it's all right for them to let go. Just take it easy and make the stretching section of your workout as serene and sensuous as you possibly can.

Stretch 1.

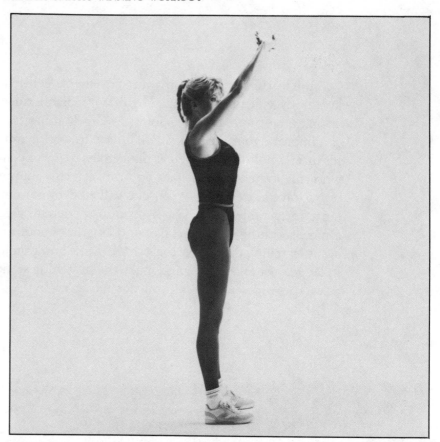

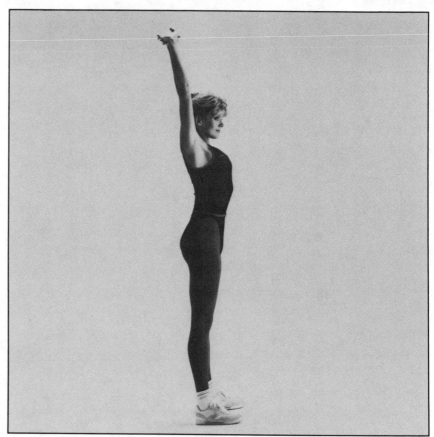

STEP 1A

Stand erect and interlace your fingers with your palms facing outward. Extend your arms forward at about a 45° angle. If you feel any back pain, bend your knees slightly.

STEP 1B

As you exhale, keep your arms straight and raise them up and back as far as you can. Hold 15 seconds.

Return to the starting position as you inhale.

★ Repeat this stretch four times ★

Stretch 2.

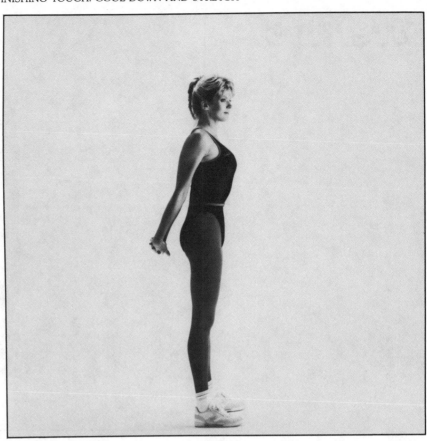

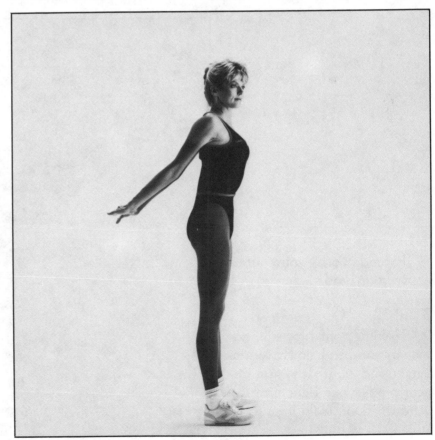

STEP 2A

Stand erect and interlace your fingers behind your hips with your palms facing up. Don't arch your back. Squeeze your buttocks, keeping your spine long.

STEP 2B

As you exhale, keep your arms straight and press them gently to the rear for 15 seconds while maintaining good posture.

Return to the starting position as you inhale.

★Repeat this stretch four times★

Stretch 3.

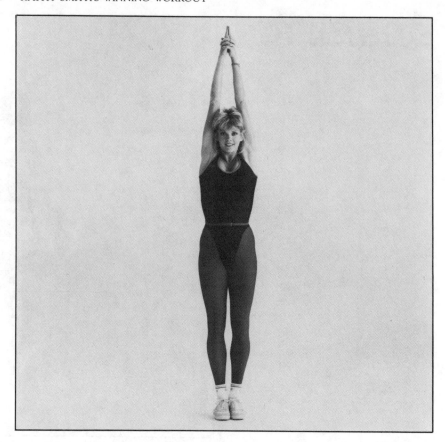

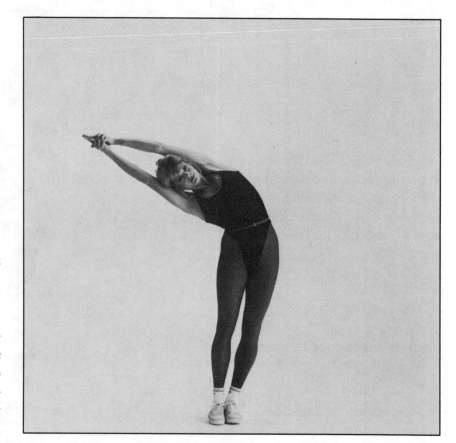

STEP 3A

Extend both your arms above your head.

STEP 3B

Holding your hips still, exhale as you bend slowly to the left, using your left arm to gently pull your right arm toward the floor. Hold in an easy stretch 15 seconds.

★Repeat this stretch four times for each side, alternating sides ★

Stretch 4.

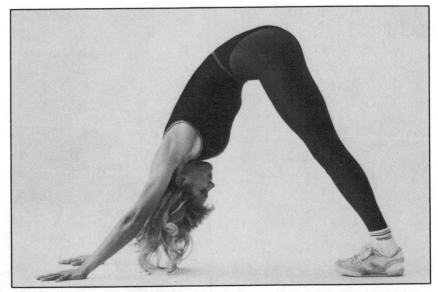

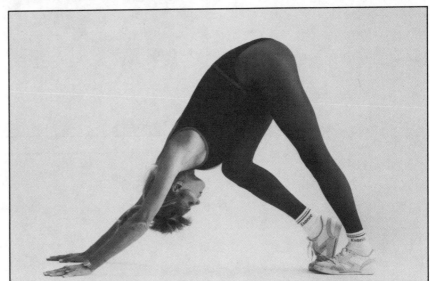

STEP 4A

Bend forward at your hips with your feet together and your hands flat on the floor. Raise your right heel and bend your right knee while keeping your left leg straight with your left heel on the floor.

Hold 15 seconds.

STEP 4B

Lower your right heel, straighten your right leg, then raise your left heel and bend your left knee, while keeping your right heel on the floor.

Hold 15 seconds.

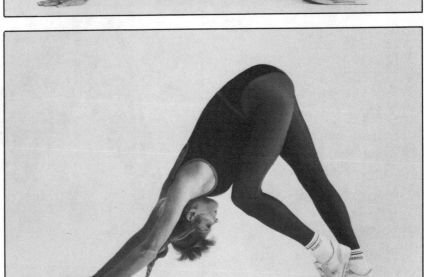

★Repeat this stretch four times★

145

Stretch 5.

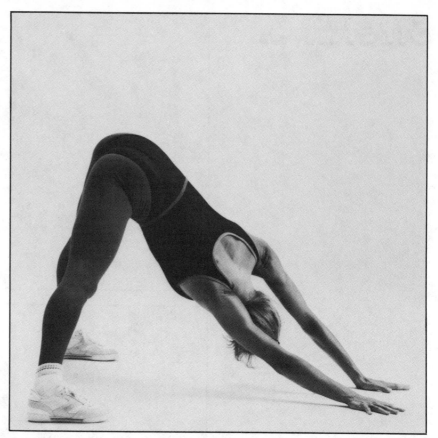

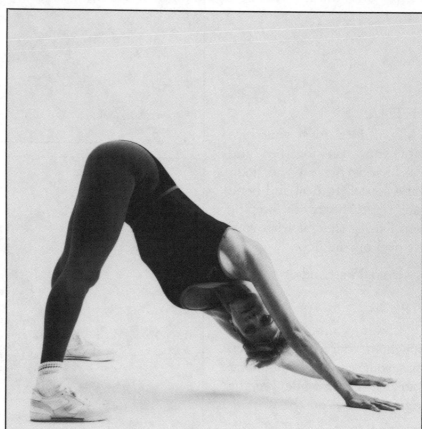

STEP 5A

Keeping your hands still, walk your feet apart and twist your upper body to the left.

Hold 15 seconds.

STEP 5B

Twist your upper body to the right.

Hold 15 seconds.

★Repeat this stretch four times★

Stretch 6.

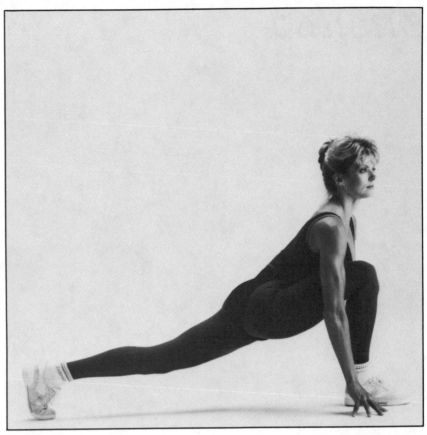

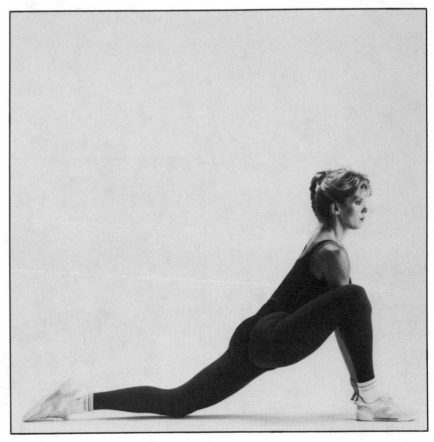

STEP 6A

Lunge forward with your right leg as far as you can and place your fingertips on the floor, on either side of your right leg.

Hold 15 seconds (no bouncing!).

STEP 6B

Maintaining your balance, drop your back knee on the floor and press your hips down and forward.

Hold 15 seconds.

★Repeat this stretch four times for each leg★

Stretch 7.

STEP 7A. The Cat Stretch.

With your legs bent under you, reach forward with your hands as far as you can and stretch your arms, shoulders, and back.

Hold 15 seconds.

STEP 7B

With your palms pressing down, pull back with your arms straight.

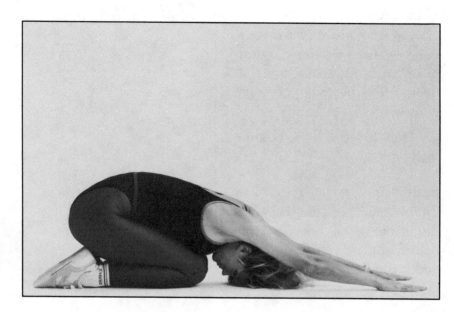

Stretch 8.

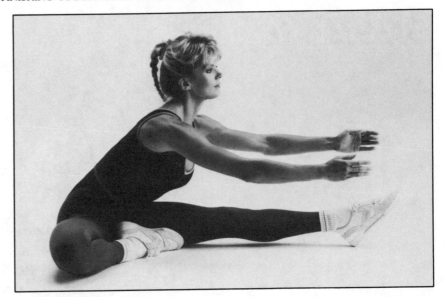

STEP 8A

Sit on the floor with one leg extended in front of you. Tuck your other foot against the inside of your extended leg. With your back flat, reach gently forward with both arms extended (no bouncing!).

Hold 15 seconds.

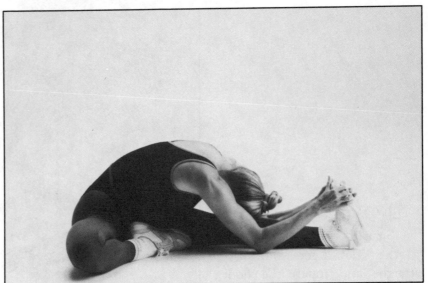

STEP 8B

Relax and round your back, bending forward as you try to grasp your foot with both hands and try to touch your forehead to your knee.

Hold 15 seconds.

STEP 8C

Slowly bring your extended leg back to the tuck position and try to touch your forehead to your feet.

Hold 15 seconds.

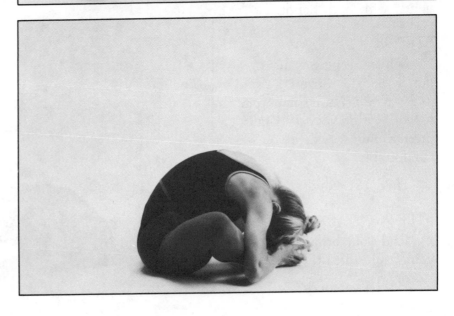

 Repeat this stretch four times for each leg, alternating legs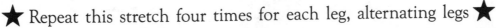

Stretch 9.

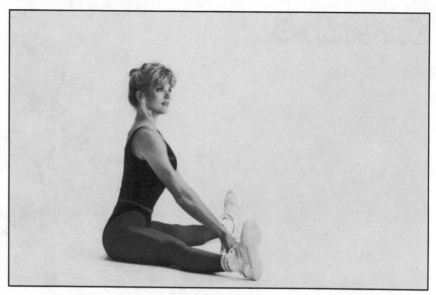

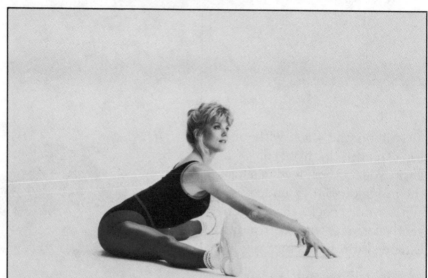

STEP 9A

Sit with your legs extended to the sides. Keep your back straight and touch the floor lightly with both hands.

STEP 9B

While keeping your back flat, walk your fingers forward as far as you can. It's important to work within your own limits. Stretch only to where you feel comfortable.

Hold 15 seconds.

STEP 9C

Fold your arms and touch your forehead to the floor.

Hold 15 seconds.

 Repeat this stretch four times

Stretch 10.

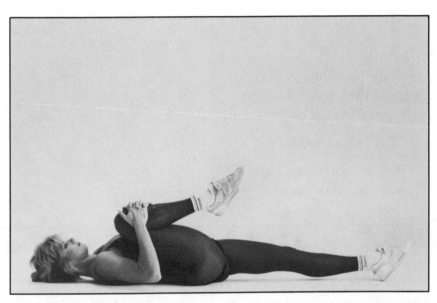

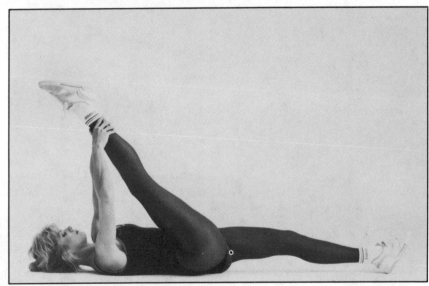

STEP 10A

Lie on your back and pull your right knee toward your chest.

Hold in an easy stretch 15 seconds.

STEP 10B

Slowly straighten your right leg and pull it toward your head (don't force).

Hold in an easy stretch 15 seconds.

 Repeat this stretch four times for each leg, alternating legs. ★

Stretch 11

STEP 11A

Lie with your hands clasped behind your head. Cross your right leg over your left leg.

Hold 15 seconds.

STEP 11B

Twist your hips to the right as far as you can while keeping your shoulders flat on the floor.

Hold 15 seconds

Repeat with your left leg crossed over your right leg.

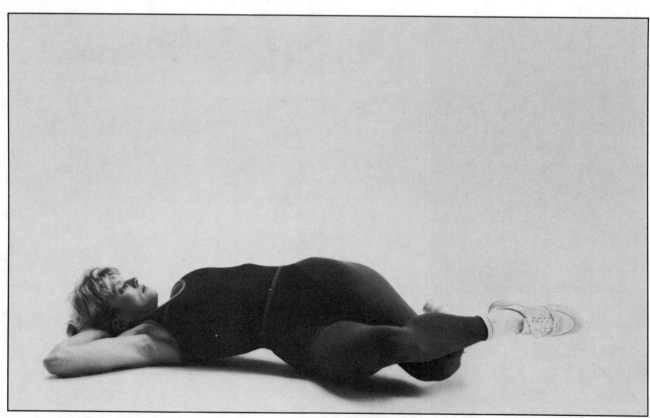

★ Repeat this stretch four times for each side, alternating sides ★

CHAPTER TEN

Finding Your Own Balance: Eating to Win

I'm not going to put you on a diet to go along with your workout program. For one thing, the very word diet—as in "starvation diet," hard-boiled-egg-and-grapefruit diet, or lose-ten-pounds-by-tomorrow-night diet —is fast becoming obsolete. Studies of perpetual dieters—that is, the overweight Americans who spend most of their lives losing weight, then gaining it right back again—have shown that radical dieting is part of the problem, not the solution.

Instant weight loss is just that—weight that's lost for about an instant. The reason: your body has a highly efficient survival mechanism that causes it to interpret any dramatic cutback in calorie consumption as a sign of impending starvation. It responds to this "threat" by slowing down your metabolism and converting every calorie you do ingest into fat and storing it away, while it burns muscle and other vital tissue for energy. When you return to your normal eating habits, your system continues to operate in the starvation mode until it seems safe to return to normal, with the result that you quickly gain back *more* than you lost. The more often you diet, the more quickly and efficiently your body slows down, locking you even more tightly into the starve-and-gain cycle.

There is a way out of the yo-yo diet syndrome, however. Regular exercise, particularly exercise with an aerobic component, has been shown to raise your basal metabolism, so that you not only burn extra calories while you work out, you also continue to burn them for up to 15 hours afterward, even when you're at rest. This is good news for women, who can't possibly get all the nutrients they need to stay healthy on the kind of 600- to 1,000-calorie-a-day diets that were the norm for so many years. And it's *great* news for anyone who's tired of feeling deprived all the time.

If you're serious about staying fit and healthy, you'll have to eat right as well as exercise. Think about it—would you spend a lot of time and money having your car tuned up, then take it out and fill the tank with soda? Of course not! Yet most people seem to expect their bodies—far more delicate mechanisms than a car engine—to run on worse fuel than that.

What, exactly, does "eating right" mean? The answer varies from individual to individual. That's the second reason for my refusal to prescribe a diet for you. I believe that the best way to find out what eating right means for you is to experiment—within balanced, nutritionally-sound limits, of course—until you find the foods that make you feel good and function best. I can't tell you what to eat; I can only tell you what I've learned from my own experience.

I've been experimenting with my own diet ever since college days, and at some point, I'll bet I tried them all: the high-protein diets, the vegetarian diets, fasting, weird foods—you name it. I made a lot of mistakes along the way. For instance, I wouldn't advise you to go on a strict vegetarian diet, as I did, without first learning everything there is to know about food combining. I was teaching aerobics at the time, and pretty soon I couldn't climb a flight of stairs after class without feeling faint. When I finally went to see my doctor, he discovered that I'd become severely anemic and lacked about half the essential nutrients I needed to stay alive—all because I'd embarked on the diet without a thorough understanding of the principles behind it.

Eventually, though, I learned through trial and error what eating right means for me. Now I aim for a balance, but a balance that works for *my* body. I follow the recent recommendations calling for a diet low in fat, consisting of about 65% carbohydrates and a moderate amount of protein. But some people can't seem to digest that much roughage easily, and if I were they, I'd look for a different (but equally sound) balance.

By now, I'm so sensitive to my body's responses to certain foods that I'm not even tempted to overindulge in them. For example, I have no particular problem with sugar. I don't crave it and I eat very little of it, but I also know that a few bites of some sweet dessert isn't going to kill me. Fats are another story—eating a high-fat meal not only makes me feel sluggish, it also makes me feel downright anxious and insecure. Because I'm tuned in to this reaction, eating a meal of greasy junk foods or rich sauces is about the least appealing prospect I can imagine. And just by avoiding those foods, while exercising and keeping the rest of my intake sensible, I'm able to maintain my ideal weight without having to count calories.

Certainly, you should follow sensible guidelines for healthy eating. Studies of very old people have shown that the most long-lived among them rarely resorted to extreme eating habits, but tended throughout their lives to eat a balanced variety of foods. The four food groups you learned about in grade school are still valid guidelines for eating right. And we know now that fresh foods are much better for you than the over-processed foods to which too many Americans have become accustomed. But within these basic guidelines, people's reactions to specific foods vary enormously, and you'll be better off if you do some careful experimenting on your own, instead of accepting someone else's formula for eating well. Your training diary can be an invaluable aid in helping you develop a sensible diet that's right for you. If you feel unusually tired, spaced-out or irritable after lunch one day, think back to what you just ate. Then glance at your records to see how you felt the last time you ate the same foods. Pretty soon, you'll begin to see correlations between your eating habits and your overall feelings of well-being. Eventually, you'll learn which foods are and which are not right for you. The more aware you become that certain foods do more than just make you fat, the more motivated you'll be to avoid them.

That's my personal formula for successful eating. Interestingly, it's backed up in a recent book called *Keeping It Off: Winning at Weight Loss*, for which authors Robert Colvin and Susan Olsen interviewed a number of people who had beaten the statistics by losing 20 pounds or more and keeping them off for at least five years. The authors wanted to know if there was a particular method or set of principles that had allowed these people to succeed where 95% of dieters fail. What they learned was that each of these formerly fat people attributed his or her success to *not* following anyone else's prescription for weight loss, but experimenting until he or she came up with a personal eating plan. Some of them had, indeed, joined weight-loss groups for a while, but used these programs mainly as sources for basic nutritional information. Then they quickly went back to the pattern of experimenting, learning from each failure and refusing to stop until they'd developed their own eating habits, ones that they felt were entirely right for them. This method, it seems, was the only one that allowed them to take responsibility for their own eating habits. In the end, taking responsibility, rather than waiting for someone else to come up with a magic formula, was their key to success.

The authors did uncover one pattern common to nearly all of their weight-loss winners, however, and it agrees so completely with my own philosophy that I'm sharing it with you in the hope that you'll try it. They found, almost without realizing it, that each of their subjects had, in his or her own idiosyncratic way, virtually eliminated sugar and fats and drastically cut salt intake. This is basically the style of eating I came up with after my own years of experimentation, too. I've found it to be not only an *effective* way to eat healthfully and control my weight, but also a very easy one; it means I don't have to walk around with a calorie counter or deprive myself of an occasional splurge. I'd like to recommend a very simple way for you to integrate these eating changes into your Winning Workout program while you continue to test a variety of eating plans.

Pick whichever of the three categories of foods—those high in sugar, fat, or salt—you think you can most easily live without. During Phase 1 of your workout program, concentrate on drastically cutting your intake of all foods in that category. You don't have to eliminate them completely; just reduce your consumption until you can honestly say you eat very little of those foods. Putting yourself on your honor is the only possible way to succeed, in this or in any other weight-loss plan. Having the body you want is, in the end, your responsibility and no one else's. If you're an avowed chocoholic, for instance, don't try to cut out sugars during Phase 1, cut down on fats or salty foods instead. Tell yourself that you'll have to reduce your intake of these foods for just four weeks, not forever, but for those four weeks, you're going to be as good as gold.

Next, pick your second problem-food category and say goodbye to it for the duration of Phase 2. Naturally, you'll be way ahead of the game if you continue to eliminate or cut down on the food category you dropped in Phase 1, but if you feel you just can't go on without eating hollandaise sauce on your eggs Benedict, go ahead and reintroduce that food category into your diet, in moderation, using the knowledge that you've lived perfectly happily without it for four weeks to help you control your consumption.

Wait until you reach Phase 3 before you tackle the food category that tends to be your diet downfall. By this time, you'll have made so much progress in your workouts that your self-esteem and self-control will be at a high point, and it will be easier for you to conquer temptation. Besides, you already will have proven to yourself that you can live without certain foods for at least a month at a time without really suffering.

The great advantage to this plan is that, by the end of 12 weeks, you'll have sharply reduced your consumption of the major contributors to overweight, without having deprived yourself of much at all. I don't believe that there are such things as "bad" foods, only foods we eat too much of, and sugar, fat, and salt are at the top of the list for Americans. Each of them, eaten in large quantities, not only makes you fat, but also contributes to long lists of debilitating and sometimes fatal diseases. How much of any of them do you really need? I'm not saying that you can't have a bite of chocolate cake, but you're not going to feel deprived if you don't eat the whole cake—you're going to feel *better*. While you're cutting down on one category, you can continue to enjoy foods from the other two. The point of the plan is to change your eating habits *a little at a time*.

Trying to alter a lifetime of eating behavior radically in a few days or a couple of weeks is the best way to insure failure. Giving yourself time to adjust to small improvements, and to become aware that they make you look and feel better, is the way to start eating right for life.

Postscript

Using Free Weights in Standard Exercise Routines

Wearing light wrist and ankle weights during an exercise class can boost the benefits you get from traditional, calisthenics-based workouts. In fact, adding weight to these workouts may be just what you need to break out of a discouraging slump, to start seeing improvement again after leveling off for a few months, or simply to beat boredom. The reason is that the same principle of progressive overload described in Chapter 5 applies to any exercise program. If you've been attending the same exercise class regularly for some time, your body (not to mention your mind) has long been adapted to the demands of your class's basic routine, and if you want to get off your present plateau, you're going to have to up the ante. The easiest way to do that, if you plan to continue with the class, is to wear one- or two-pound weights on your wrists and/or ankles when you perform the exercises.

Keep in mind that not everyone should wear ankle or wrist weights, and they're not equally suited to every exercise. If you're out of shape, have a great deal of weight to lose, or are just beginning an exercise program, the basic exercises done *without* weights will probably provide more than enough challenge for you. Only when you've lost weight or become fit enough to feel that your current exercise program is too easy should you try adding weights.

Avoiding violent, bouncing movements is even more important when you wear ankle or wrist weights. It's virtually impossible to maintain correct form during violent movements, and you'll end up putting unnecessary strain on your joints and ligaments. Check with your instructor that the exercises you do in class can be done safely and effectively while wearing weights.

One last point: look for weights that have no bulky closures to rub or chafe your skin, and make sure the weights fit snugly enough so that they won't slide around on your wrists or ankles when you move; this is not only uncomfortable, it also can throw off your balance enough to undermine the effects of the exercise.

By the way, you can help condition your muscles by wearing your ankle and wrist weights while you perform ordinary household chores or go for a walk. Needless to say, you won't turn into Miss Universe just by wearing weights while you vacuum, but every little bit helps.